Kiss From A Rose

Natasha Vince

authorHOUSE®

AuthorHouse™
1663 Liberty Drive
Bloomington, IN 47403
www.authorhouse.com
Phone: 1-800-839-8640

First published by AuthorHouse   06/21/2011

ISBN: 978-1-4567-8253-5 (sc)

Printed in the United States of America

I am a 25-year-old graduate from Warwick University. I graduated with a 2.1 in Comparative American Studies in summer 2009, and currently work for Sky News.

The novel is an account of my experience of having cancer over the last ten years. It is very personal, and very honest. It focuses mainly on my initial diagnoses at the age of 16, but also touches on my four subsequent relapses. I wrote it primarily for other teenagers who are about to go through similar treatment, those who are beginning their journey, and perhaps facing months of chemotherapy and radiotherapy. I hope I have been successful in my design for the novel to be eye opening, but not daunting, comforting, but not sugarcoated.

I live in Kent, surrounded by a very supportive family. My boyfriend of four years has also shown unfaltering strength throughout my battle with the disease, he has been a pillar of strength during my darkest hours.

'Kiss From A Rose' is about appreciating the beauty of life's bud as it blooms. Although you may catch yourself on life's thorns, the pain you incur does not make the rose any less exquisite.

In Memory of my Beloved Grandad.
A True Gentleman.

And Debra Booth.
Pricked by similar thorns to mine, her rose has bloomed.

A beautiful rose, life blossoms with each year that passes us by. But some things are sent to try us. Although when they prick, the thorns in our lives sting and cause us pain, it is these imperfections, which we must accept as a part of life, that makes each flower that little bit more spectacular.

N.V.

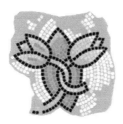

As I sit waiting for the phone call, I reflect on my journey so far. I think of the good times, the holidays I've had with my family, the memories I have made with my friends; I realise that I've had a good 25 years. But I've also tasted my fair share of pain. Life is as precious, as fragile and as beautiful as a rose; yet the thorns on my rose have caused much anguish in recent years. As I sit by the phone I'm frightened I'm about to feel their sting all over again.

Although it has repeatedly tried to suffocate and strangle the life from my rose bud, I have battled hard to overcome the fate that cancer all too often brings to many; I'm not sure of how much fight I have left in me. It is days like these when I am expecting news about my scans that I realise what a lonely disease cancer is. Although I have many friends and so much love and support from my family, nobody truly knows how I feel. Nobody knows what's going on in my head, no one can really understand the torment I put myself through throughout the days leading up to hearing the results. And I wouldn't want them to. But this has been my life for the past ten years, living with this dark shadow looming over me so often blocking the sunlight from my rose. It has been two years since I last needed treatment, and although it is normal procedure to visit my consultant to pick up my results after routine scans, often now he spares me the journey by phoning me instead. So today, while I sit and wait for the call from my consultant which will reveal the results of my latest scan, I struggle to justify the pain I'll need to suffer in order to get better if I'm told I'll need more treatment. I wonder will it all be worth it. The agony, the fear, the isolation. After five diagnoses, is it finally time to give in, to allow my rose to succumb to this poison? Maybe. Maybe it would be easier to let go while my body surrenders under attack. But then again, I have so much to live for . . . .

As It Was In The Beginning

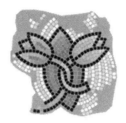

The year was 2001, I was 15 and life was good. My rose bud was blooming, with not too many thorns pricking along the way. I had friendships that I thought would last a lifetime, a boyfriend, Pete, who I was infatuated with, and I was doing pretty well at school. My best friend, Lucy, I had known since we were five. We met each other at Rainbows—like Brownies, but for tiny people. I have beautiful memories of us hunting for Easter eggs in the mild spring evenings together, and comparing our simple ballet dance routines. But our lives soon took us in separate directions. Her parents sent her to a private primary school, and with my mum being on her own bringing up my younger brother and I, I went to our local Catholic school.

It was there I met four of the most important people in my life. Rebecca, Katharine, Louise and Justine. My best friends; my soul mates. There's nothing we wouldn't do for each other; no secrets we would keep from each other, nothing we didn't know about each other. My time at primary school was carefree, fun and full of adventure—everything childhood should be. And so I was growing up. Life went pretty smoothly throughout my younger years, although it was just my mum who brought us up, we have always been close to my grandparents. Spoiling us at every opportunity, treating us to unbeatable fun-packed holidays on the coast every year, they soon helped me to forget the pain of catching myself on life's first thorn, which developed the day my dad left us. I was five. I guess I'll never get over the day he drove away; the day he turned his back on us and started a new life with a new family. So easy, it seems that he could walk away, though I still have no idea why. The years have since soothed the pain of that thorn, and under the guidance of a huge, loving, generous family, my rose continued to bloom.

I lost touch with my primary school friends for a short while when we left to go to Secondary school, it was a shame, but I guess life takes you on different paths, so that when you meet up again you can share your experiences and teach each other the lessons you've learnt along the way. But it was at this new school that I crossed paths again with my Rainbows buddy Lucy. We weren't in the same class initially, but as we approached our GCSEs we picked a couple of the same subjects, so were put together for a few classes such as Music and English. We soon became inseparable, we were best friends and did everything together. We attended a few out-of-school clubs relating to music, so we pretty much lived in each other's pockets! I knew who she fancied, she knew who I liked, we did our homework together, we even recorded a duet together for our music class! If only we'd known about Simon Cowell then, we could have been the next Beyonce and Lady Gaga! Wishful thinking! I think we were more like the Cheeky Girls whenever we warbled together! After a turbulent few years of finding my feet and a nice bunch of girls to mix with, I was really starting to enjoy school. As well as Lucy, I had a good group of friends and we did what every other group of teenage girls did: shopped, gossiped and giggled over boys.

The year of our GCSEs was approaching, and we were dreading the exams. We soon began to look forward to the summer holidays when they would be out of the way, and we would be free! My 16th birthday fell right in the middle of the exams, so mum suggested I throw a huge party after them to celebrate my birthday, and to mark the beginning of a new era for everyone. As the exams grew closer we were all feeling the pressure and stressing over getting all our coursework completed on time, of course, we all left everything to the very last minute. I remember sitting up until four o' clock in the morning with my mum the night before my music composition deadline, trying to record my 'masterpiece' on a child's recording machine. All of our coursework, including the composition was due in around the time we were sitting our mock exams. Although I had been studying hard for the mocks, I really wanted to do well in my coursework—especially music. I play three instruments piano, violin and the flute, and play each quite well, so thought this would be my strongest subject. I thought I was really prepared for it.

Like everyone else, I left much of the actual composing right up until the final week before it had to be submitted. Despite this, however, I thought I was being ultra-organised when I downloaded some software, which recorded the music you composed from the computer onto a CD. This was exciting stuff, as recording CDs had not been around for long then, and so I felt immeasurably tech-savvy. Yes, I thought I was really on top of things, however, events were not to run smoothly for me the night before my deadline. Despite numerous checks to ensure the software was definitely working, for some reason when I really needed it, it refused to behave! Nothing would record on the CD, I tried over and over again, but each time the CD came out blank. After several hours of panicking, and threatening to throw the computer out of the window, I sat and stared at my beautiful manuscript on the monitor screen, devastated that it would never now fall upon and delight the ears of my fellow classmates. I wasn't sure what I was going to do, it was far too late to call one of my friends and ask them for help, and I started to panic. Just as I was threatening to give up the music GCSE completely, mum had an ingenious idea. She ran to get a toy recording machine Dominic and I both used to play with when we were younger. She climbed up into the loft and I heard her scuffling around for ages until she emerged and descended upon the landing triumphantly, with the little 'Trust Tomy' toy in her hand. Trust Tomy indeed! The machine had a tiny microphone device built into it, and so I held it up to the speaker on the computer as my composition rang out. I recorded the piece onto a tape in the tiny machine, and as this was a time before MP3 players and the like, a tape was still absolutely sufficient technology to hand in to my music teacher! When the music stopped ringing out from the computer speakers, I rewound the tape and prayed that it had recorded. Sure enough the little toy machine played out my music loud and clear, and mum and I danced around the room to it in celebration. It was about four in the morning by now; the neighbours must have thought we were absolutely insane, and my brother was killing himself laughing as he watched us. We were both drained and exhausted, and mum was covered in dust from going through years of memories in the loft to find the recorder. I couldn't believe that when all the latest technology failed, this tiny piece of old plastic, which hadn't seen the light of day for years, pulled through for me! I'll never forget the way my mum helped me that night, how she stayed up with me and searched with such determination for the little recording device so that I wouldn't throw all of my hard work away. But little did I know that that was just the tip of the iceberg when it came to her giving me unquestioning support and understanding.

Thankfully, completing the rest of my coursework was less eventful, and I could now concentrate on my mocks.

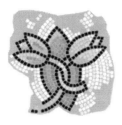

As we sat in a classroom in complete silence, I turned over the first page of the mock exam paper I was dreading the most. I really struggled with maths, but I'd had a good and supportive teacher, so wanted to do both her and myself proud. I flicked through the rest of the paper, checking to make sure that it wasn't going to be a complete disaster, before turning back to the front page breathing a small sigh of relief. Suddenly a huge burst of pain seared through my stomach; I thought I was going to faint. The pain was so intense, I began sweating, and I could feel a pulse beating against the inside of my head. I doubled over holding my tummy, praying that, this time, it would pass quickly. You see, it wasn't the first time this pain had struck me. I had been suffering from these severe stomach cramps for around six months, I had been to see my GP countless times, and each visit saw him prescribe me stronger painkillers. In his infinite wisdom, he took the easy option of diagnosing the pain as menstrual cramps, but I knew my body. I'd been having periods for a few years by then, and they had never been as bad as this. Each time I saw the doctor, I insisted that it was nothing to do with my periods; the pain was constant, not simply for one week of the month. It was such an intense pain, that I physically wanted to rip my stomach out; I wanted to scream with the agony, I wanted to punch and kick until somebody would listen. Every time I entered the doctor's surgery, I felt like I was screaming in the dark with no one to help me; and the one person who had the power to do anything for me was not only deaf to my cries, he was turning a blind eye to my suffering as well. He made me feel pathetic, he made me feel that I was complaining about something that every woman on the planet copes with every month for the majority of their lives. He made me feel like a silly little girl, taking up his valuable time with my trivial grumbling.

So I tried to carry on with my life. My boyfriend and I decided to cool things down between us until after all the exams. I said it was a good idea because as well as my GCSEs, he had his A levels to study for and besides, we'd have many good times to look forward to once the stress and pressure of exams had passed. I soon completed my mocks and began preparing for the real thing! After being misdiagnosed at the GP's surgery so many times, I began to believe that perhaps the cramps really *were* just bad period pains, and that I was going to have to live with the pain for the next 40 years. I thought I may as well get used to it, and get on with it. But over time, the pain intensified even more. It was constant, and though I was trying to live with it, I couldn't ignore it for much longer. The cramps would seize me throughout the day and, as my GCSEs were approaching, they were making it increasingly difficult for me to concentrate and retain information. Maths and science were not my strongest subjects at the best of times, but I was struggling to grasp new, simple concepts. As I felt I was falling behind, I began to lose interest in class, devoting all my attention and willpower trying to overcome the pain that was engulfing me.

As well as my concentration, I gradually began losing my appetite too. Soon, I physically couldn't eat. Every time I attempted a meal, I felt full almost immediately. I remember one occasion, my nan had prepared a full roast dinner for the family, having worked hard all morning preparing a feast for us, all I could manage was literally a small roast potato, before I had to dash to the loo to be sick. After a while people around me began to think I had an eating disorder. It was true, I was losing a dramatic amount of weight, and fast, but it certainly wasn't through choice. I wanted to eat, I wanted to feel normal, I wanted to sit down and enjoy a complete meal with my family, but it was impossible for me. The thought of dinner, and lunch times in the school canteen filled me with dread, as I could hear the girls who were supposed to be my friends talking about me. They thought I wasn't eating in order to get attention, they thought I was being pathetic and self-absorbed. They couldn't have been more wrong.

Sitting in the Biology class, I heard my stomach roar, and I just couldn't understand how I was obviously so hungry, yet felt so full all the time. Soon, I could feel my teachers running out of patience with me too. I'm sure many of them also thought my behaviour was a result of a craving for attention; attending an all girls' school, I think it is fair to say that all of us were very conscious of our appearance. Being slim and trim was at the top of everyone's list of priorities. But I was too skinny; at 5ft 4inches my weight dropped quickly to 7 stone. In the meantime, my trips to the doctor's surgery became a frequent event, each time he sent me away with bigger, stronger painkillers; each time throwing me a more irritated look as I left his office.

After months of being turned away, not being able to eat and walking around holding my stomach, I starting to think that I must be going mad. If the doctor could find nothing wrong with me, there must have been nothing wrong, so what was going on in my head that was making me think I was in all this pain? I spent every lunchtime in the school's medical room, silently crying, wishing the agony away. One morning, I was at school in the canteen, it was coming to the end of morning break, so everyone was finishing off their food and getting ready to head to their next class of the morning. There were two bells that rang at the end of each break; the first was to let you know that break was over. It told you to go to the loo and get any books or equipment you might need for your next lesson from your locker. The second rang five minutes later and indicated that you should, by now, be in the classroom ready to start the lesson. My friends and I were sitting chatting at a table quite near to the entrance door to the canteen as the first bell rang, we all stood up and gathered our things together. Suddenly the pain stuck again, and I doubled over clutching my tummy. I stood bent over the table wincing in agony as the rest of the school bustled past me. There were two teachers on duty in the food hall that morning; one was the music teacher. Despite my love for music my music teacher and I didn't see eye to eye too often, she was always making patronising and degrading comments to everyone, so when we weren't in the classroom I avoided her as much as possible. As I held onto the edges of the table that morning, waiting for the pain to pass, the other teacher on duty came up and put his hand on my back and rubbed it. He looked at my music teacher asking if it was period pains, "Supposedly", she replied. "Natasha, stop moaning and get out of the bloody way! You're blocking the whole canteen! Stop complaining and get to class". I couldn't even look up at her, and practically crawled out of the food hall to my next lesson, the pain was so intense.

But now, along with the pain, I could feel a strange movement inside my tummy. Sometimes it was so violent, I can only describe it as what I imagine an expectant mother feels when her baby is kicking inside her. I was scared; I knew something was very wrong, yet still no one was listening. Soon, it became too much. Sitting in the medical room once again, I couldn't hold it in any more and I screamed. I screamed so loud until someone heard me. Until someone really heard me. Until someone helped me.

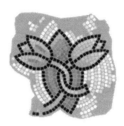

I remember the head teacher running down the corridor almost skidding into the medical room. Her name was Mrs Hutchinson, and fantastic at her job, she wanted the best for all her pupils but wasn't afraid to put us in our place when we needed it! The look on her face as she met me in the medical room that lunchtime was a mixture of fear, confusion and concern. She tried to calm me down, but I was in agony. I didn't want anyone to touch me; I didn't want anyone to hold me. I was sweating, crying and retching. I couldn't breath, I couldn't move with the pain. The school office called my mum. She was at work a good 40 minutes drive away; but it took her less than 20 minutes to get to me. She was working in a primary school in Sidcup as a Nursery Teacher at the time, so would have had to find someone to look after her class before she even left her school. She got to me as quickly as she could, although to me it felt like hours. When she arrived she burst through the front doors, grabbed me, and rushed me to our local hospital, Queen Mary's in Sidcup. She later told me that the journey there was like being in a car with the girl from the film, 'The Exorcist'. I have no memory of the journey, but she often teases me as she recalls me screaming and swearing at her. Normally, I wouldn't dream of speaking to my mum like this, I'd get a thick lip if I was that cheeky! But I think she made an exception on this occasion! As I was in so much pain I was running a temperature, so suddenly started taking my clothes off in the car, by the time we reached the hospital I was exhausted, frightened and practically naked!

I was taken to a bed in the children's department in A&E of Queen Mary's, and was left lying there for a couple of hours until a doctor became free to examine me. Due to the pain and my description of movement within my tummy, the medical staff obviously assumed I was pregnant. I was 15 and the school I attended, Townley Grammar, had a bit of a reputation. It was an all girls' school, and we were collectively called the 'Townley Tarts' by pupils in other schools in the area. General opinion was that we concentrated more on boys, than our school work, so my protests of not being pregnant fell on deaf ears! I tried to explain that unless it was the result of divine intercession and this was a second immaculate conception, there was absolutely no way I could be pregnant. However, they went ahead with a pregnancy test 'just to be safe'. I remember my mum, Mary, telling me to just be honest, she told me that if I was pregnant to just say so, and we could deal with it together. I started laughing. I was in absolute agony and couldn't believe no one was listening. But I could see how worried my mum was; in her eyes, being 15 and pregnant was not the life she had hoped for her daughter, but then at least there would have been an explanation for the pain. The medical team looking after me went on to carry out five further pregnancy tests, convinced that eventually one would show up positive, and the pain I was in would prove to be the result of complications. However, just as I had told them countless times, as each test came back negative they soon came round to the idea that I actually wasn't pregnant! So, the experts once again diagnosed bad period pains. A gynaecologist made a quick visit; he didn't even examine me, but simply prescribed more painkillers and sent me home.

The medication he gave me must have been quite strong as it knocked me out for the rest of the afternoon, and brought some much welcome rest. I woke later in the evening to the sharp pain that was all too familiar to me.

The effectiveness of the gynaecologist's painkillers quickly diminished, and once again nothing was helping to numb the agony I was in. I continued going to school for the rest of the week; I tried so hard to attend all my classes and concentrate despite my extreme discomfort. However, by the end of the week, I was back in the medical room, with the office staff again frantically trying to get hold of my mum. As my head teacher came in to sit with me while mum was on her way, I rocked on the edge of the bed to try to ease the pain. Looking back I realise how much time she spent with me, and how she was the only one in that school who really did believe that I was in pain. When many other teachers lost patience with me, and accused me of being dramatic and seeking attention, she didn't. And when I look back at all those times she sat with me in that tiny room by the school office, I see the genuine helplessness in her eyes. As I left school to make yet another trip to the A&E department in Queen Mary's hospital she told my mum to refuse to leave until they found out exactly what was wrong. And that's exactly what mum did.

The hospital staff must have seen me coming; the moody teenager who couldn't cope with a few period pains was back, and screaming the place down once again. My grandad also turned up, and with him my brother, Dominic had finished school for the day, and my grandad had picked him up before coming to the hospital to see if I was alright. They both looked terrified. I was screaming, and again, I was trying to take off as many layers of clothing as possible because I was so hot. Dominic tried to hold my hand, but I shook him away, he stood looking at me helplessly, the tears streaming down his face. As I lay on the hospital bed in just my pants, tights and bra, my grandad ran around A&E desperately trying to get a nurse or a doctor to take the pain away and stop me from crying. This time they gave me no pregnancy tests, but they did give me an X-ray. The scan showed that I was extremely congested, so they suggested I took some strong laxatives and be on my way. But my mum could see that it was more than that. She wanted an explanation as to why I could be so congested that I could only manage a roast potato at dinner before running to the toilet to throw up. Why hadn't my system sorted itself out by now? This had been going on for almost a year; it wasn't normal. Surely there must be something blocking my insides to make my condition so severe, but nobody had any answers for her; instead they formed a new theory as to what the problem was. I had been assigned a consultant in the A&E department, and he had requested the X-ray, for which I was grateful, but an X-ray can only show up so much. It doesn't provide a detailed image of tissues and organs, and so it had missed the extent of the problem. He told my mum he believed that I was in a certain amount of discomfort due to the congestion in my intestines, however, the intense pain I was complaining of, he believed, was simply in my head. He told her I was attention seeking and doing my best to get out of my upcoming GCSEs. He suggested that she take me home and administer some discipline around the house, to ensure that I no longer persisted in such juvenile behaviour. He also advised that she take me to a psychologist, because if I wanted to get out of a few exams this badly, I clearly had some underlying behavioural problems. I lay on the hospital bed in the foetal position, clutching my stomach, listening to an educated professional telling me I was going mad. Seeing me shake with the pain, a nurse brought over some gas 'n' air. I grabbed hold of the mask, clutching it to my mouth as I closed my eyes and threw myself into darkness. I lay there praying to die. In front of me I could see a skull and crossbones, a bit like on the Jolly Roger flag, but there was no sea, no ocean breeze, no boat to take me away from here. The skull and crossbones remained flying for a while. I thought if death was the only way to escape this agony, then I would welcome it with open arms, I didn't feel an ounce of guilt or fear. Listening to the doctor, my mum was infuriated. She knew how hard I worked at school, the determination I had shown not to let myself fall behind despite the pain I was in, and how badly I wanted to succeed and do well in my exams. But as always, she retained her dignity, thanked the 'professional' for his advice and agreed to act upon it. However, before we left, she tactfully asked that he give me an ultrasound scan, just to put her mind at rest. To this day, I have no idea what made her ask for this specific scan, I also have no idea why he agreed—to shut me up perhaps, to finally be able to close my file. But in that moment, mum saved my life.

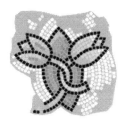

By now, I had been put on a ward to free up some space in A&E following my X-ray, so I was temporarily considered an in-patient. As a result, the ultrasound was booked and carried out almost immediately, if I had still been in A&E I would have been waiting for hours yet. By this point I had given up hope of the pain ever going away, I lay in the darkness in the scanning room still wanting it all to just stop. I wanted to let go, exhausted from the pain, and the battle of getting people to listen to me. I thought to myself, if that was the only way this pain was going to go away, then I was ready. As the radiographer made herself comfortable, I winced in pain as she covered me in lubricating jelly and gently placed the probe onto my tummy. The scan was quick, it was over within a few minutes. I assumed this was because, as before, they could see nothing wrong and were ready to give me my marching orders, with the expectation of seeing me back in A&E the following week. But I was wrong. She turned to me and said, "My God girl. You must be in absolute agony". I thought I was hearing things. I looked at her; a wave of confusion overwhelmed me, did someone finally believe me? She explained that something was blocking my large intestine, to the extent that it was twisted so badly it was no longer in its usual place. She showed me the screen, and I saw my bowel contracting and moving around my abdomen trying to push whatever was blocking it, out. This explained the strange kicking sensations I could feel in my stomach. The wave of relief that rushed over me was unimaginable; finally they could give me the correct medication, I could get out of here and crack on with passing those exams! But the radiographer's face told me things were not going to be that straightforward. She told me I needed surgery immediately, and although she couldn't tell from the scan exactly what it was that was blocking my bowel, from the size of it, it was clear that my condition was very serious.

I was rushed back to my ward to prepare for surgery and waiting for me by my bed was a surgeon and his team. He explained again that it was difficult to tell exactly what the problem was, but that I would certainly need surgery. He hurriedly explained the dangers of having an operation and presented my mum with a consent form, asking her to sign it. She took it from him, shaking, and looked at me as she said, "What do you think honey?" At 15, I couldn't give permission for them to operate myself, I was too young, so as my guardian, the responsibility fell to mum. After all this time she wanted so much for this pain to stop, but hesitated signing the form as the surgeon continued speaking. As part of the legal requirement before performing an operation, he was explaining to me all the possible things that could go wrong while I was in surgery: loss of blood; anaesthetic overdose; allergic reactions to any medicine they administered to me whilst I was under. He was basically detailing all the possible scenarios that could cause death during an operation. But he also explained that without the operation, whatever was blocking my system could erupt, or poison my body, and kill me anyway. So what choice did I have? I was terrified. I was too young to smoke, too young to drink, couldn't vote, drive or have sex, but as mum waited for me to give my permission for her to give *her* permission, I felt like she was literally signing my life away as he pushed the document in front of us and handed mum a pen. It was all happening too quickly, I had never needed an operation before other than to remove my tonsils! I was so terrified, I found myself longing for those painkillers again.

Just as I was about to go down to theatre, the surgeon asked if he could perform an internal examination, and I agreed to what was probably the most degrading moment of my life. I had an entire team of medical students around me, eager to be the first to diagnose my ailment, and impress the teacher. When he had finished, I felt an awful sensation and I turned around in the bed, horrified at the thought that I may have messed myself. I was mortified, but relieved to see from the clean sheets that I had retained a small amount of dignity. I lay back on the bed, my mum holding my hand, tears streaming down her face. I said goodbye to Dominic and to my grandad, then they wheeled me straight to theatre. The anaesthetist was kind as she explained that I would slowly feel drowsy until I eventually fell asleep. She told me to give my mum a kiss, and I'd be awake in 'recovery' in no time. But I was scared, and I could tell by the look in mum's eyes that she feared I wouldn't be waking up in 'recovery'; that I wouldn't be waking up at all. I had no words to say to her other than, "I love you, thank you for believing me. You were the only one". And with that, I closed my eyes.

21

I'll never forget the feeling waking up from that operation. I felt nothing. I felt no pain, no discomfort. For the first time in months I felt so calm, so peaceful and rested. On reflection I'm sure I must have been slightly uncomfortable from the surgery, but at the time I couldn't feel it. Compared to the agony I fell asleep in, a few stitches was absolutely nothing. Back on the ward, the hospital staff told me I would remain under hospital care for around a month, and advised my mum that she arrange my GSCEs for the following September. But I felt so great, I couldn't justify putting off the exams, and didn't want to be stuck at home revising while my friends were all out enjoying the sun! So I was up and out of that bed within the week, I just couldn't believe how great I felt. The surgeon was impressed at the speed I had recovered, and allowed me to be discharged. I booked a routine follow up appointment for a month's time to discuss the operation, but I wasn't concerned. I was told that the pain had been caused by a mass of cells, which had gathered together and blocked my large intestine. It had caused my gut to twist and that was why I couldn't eat without feeling full immediately. He said it had been completely removed, and everything was now absolutely fine. So I didn't give the follow-up appointment a second thought; how could anything be wrong, when I felt so well?

I went back to school the following Monday, and threw myself into my studies. I couldn't believe how great I felt, the difference was indescribable. After living with the pain for the last couple of years, I would often forget that it was all over and I would sit wondering when the next rush of pain was going to engulf me, but it never came. Waking up in the morning and not trying to use the loo for almost an hour before having to give up, and the luxury of eating a full meal without having to stop after few mouthfuls before trying to throw up because I felt so full, was such a novelty. I couldn't believe how fantastic it was just to feel normal, I felt alive again, that dark cloud of fear and desperation, and the longing to let go had lifted and I was me again. My exams were only a few weeks away, and I was determined to do well. There was no more pain, no more distraction, things were going my way from now on.

"Man is harder than iron, stronger than a stone and more fragile than a Rose"

Turkish Proverb

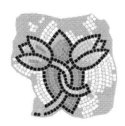

On the morning of my first exam I was so nervous, I could barely breathe. But it was English, my favourite subject, it was probably the best one to take first, to ease my mind into exam mode! I was right; after I had completed English, the next few exams didn't seem so daunting. I felt prepared and ready as I entered the exam hall at the start of each one, and elated as I ran out of the hall at the end! But after a week packed full of exams, I was looking forward to a few days break before my next scheduled exam, and nearly forgot that my follow up appointment was also due on the first of my free days. The weather was starting to improve, soon the exams would be over, I had never felt better. I was looking forward to my party exactly a week after the final exam was scheduled, and even more excited to be seeing my boyfriend, Pete, regularly again.

The day of my hospital appointment soon arrived. It was my first exam-free day, and all I wanted was to snuggle up in bed for the morning and enjoy the fact I hadn't woken up surrounded by revision papers and last minute attempts at brain cramming! Mum brought me in a cup of tea, and had run me a bath, but I was still Little Miss Grumpy as I sleepily found my way to the bathroom. I had been scheduled to attend the follow-up appointment at Queen Mary's hospital where the operation had taken place, but a few days before I was due to meet the surgeon again, we received a letter saying my local hospital had referred me to a more specialised hospital in London, but it gave no further explanation. I really couldn't understand why we had to visit another hospital, especially one so far away. I felt fine, was getting on with life, and really wanted to stay in bed! I had forgotten all about those dark days, they seemed so far away now, but mum insisted, so we went. My nan came along too, just for a day out while grandad drove us the ten minute journey from our house to Sidcup station, and he told mum to call him when we wanted to be picked up later in the day. The hospital we were going to was called the Royal Marsden, which is situated in South Kensington. I had no idea what the hospital specialised in, and had absolutely no reason to expect that things would turn out to be so serious. On the train journey I was relaxed, mum told me how nice that area of London was, and what the houses were like there, so much so that after a while, I was actually quite looking forward to getting there and having a look around! The journey wasn't a long one, and soon we were walking out of South Kensington tube station into the glorious summer sunshine. Immediately, I thought how mum had been right about the houses, as we walked along a side street that led to the hospital, I was in a daze looking at all the really fancy buildings and apartments, which were complimented by the stunning cars parked outside them!

The weather was absolutely gorgeous. The sun was beaming down on us, and I was looking forward to getting home and spending the afternoon in the garden, albeit revising! We entered the hospital, and I remember thinking how grand it was, it was completely different from Queen Mary's in Sidcup, there were even carpets along the corridors! We found the department I needed and signed in at reception. I had brought a few magazines to read while I was waiting, but needn't have bothered as I was called into the consultant's office almost as soon as I sat down. Nan stayed in the waiting room as mum and I walked down the tiny corridor, which led to the doctor's office. Inside a nurse was waiting for me, she had a sympathetic smile and beckoned me to sit on the chair next to her, she explained that the consultant would be along in a minute and asked how I was. I started gushing about my exams, how well they were going, that I was looking forward to throwing a huge party in a few weeks, and which A levels I had picked for the following September. She said nothing, she just sat looking at me with the same smile as I went on and on. Just then, an elderly, grey-haired man popped his head around the door, "Natasha?" he asked.

"Yes", I replied.

He stood with the door open, his hand remained resting on the handle as he said simply, "Because your tumour was malignant, you're going to need six months of chemo, with additional treatment if necessary". And with that, he disappeared. He came and went so fast, I had absolutely no idea what he said.

I looked at the nurse and said, "Right, is that it then?" and stood up to leave. She looked at me, with such a serious expression, she asked me if I knew what 'malignant' meant. I didn't, but from the look on her face I could tell it wasn't good news. I gave a nervous laugh, and sat back down as I said "No". I turned and looked at mum, tears were streaming down her face.

"My little honey, he's saying it was cancer" mum said. But that's ridiculous, I thought, I'm far too young for any of that, it had been my 16th birthday just a couple of days previously, mum was obviously mistaken. I looked at the nurse waiting for her to correct my mum, saying it was actually something much less serious than cancer, but she said nothing, she just looked at me with that same stupid smile. I couldn't speak, I couldn't breathe; I just couldn't take in what they were saying to me. I just sat staring at the wall behind the nurse unable to even think clearly. Suddenly, the hospital's fire alarm sounded. It was loud and constant, drilling right into my head.

"We have to evacuate", the nurse said as she jumped up.

"What? But it'll just be a practise drill won't it?" I exclaimed, "I can't go anywhere until someone tells me more about this".

"I don't know if it's a drill, that's the whole point, we need to leave the building", the nurse said getting impatient with me. I felt like I was in a dream. I couldn't believe they had just dropped this bombshell on me, and then expected me to press some sort of pause button on my emotions as we adhered to a fire-drill dress rehearsal. I felt myself standing up, and being guided by my mum towards the office door. We walked through the waiting room where we met my nan, and the three of us followed the fire escape route to the front of the hospital. There was a large crowd and three fire engines, with firemen everywhere. I was so confused. Everything was happening in slow motion, I was screaming inside, trying to wake myself up from a nightmare I just didn't see coming. My nan looked at mum, as we stood amongst the confused crowd that had assembled in the street outside the hospital.

"Everything ok?" nan asked, "this is all a bit exciting isn't it? I can't see any smoke though, can you?"

"It's cancer", mum said, disbelief in her voice. "She's got cancer".

"What?" My nan stood with a completely bewildered look on her face, "what are you talking about?" We stood in silence for a few minutes, I don't think any of us really knew what to say. "Well how serious is it? What are they going to do for her?" my nan asked.

"I don't know", mum replied, "we didn't get that far". Again, silence fell over the three of us. Mum held my hand as we stood watching the three fire engines and their crew act out their battle against a non-existent blaze until everybody was told that it was safe to re-enter the building. Mum and I were directed straight back into the consultant's room where we were joined again by the nurse, and also the doctor I had briefly met earlier. The nurse must have approached him and asked him to come back in to see us, after the outrageously inappropriate way he had addressed me. He apologised for the way he had broken the news, saying he thought I had already been made aware of the diagnosis. I still thought his attitude was rather blasé nonetheless. He explained that a biopsy had been carried out on the mass of cells that had been removed from my intestines by the doctors at Queen Mary's, and they had suspected that the cells were cancerous, forming what was called a Ewing Sarcoma. This had been confirmed by medics at the Royal Marsden, which turned out to be a hospital that specialises in 'Oncology', or cancer research and treatment. It is a rare form of the disease that is usually found in young men, normally in their legs. The doctor went on to explain that my tumour could have started anywhere before travelling around my body until it eventually got stuck in my intestine. It had done so much damage, and he predicted from the size of it that if nothing had been done, I probably wouldn't have lasted much longer than three days. Three days! I looked at mum, so grateful to her for standing her ground in Queen Mary's Hospital that day. The consultant continued by explaining that I would need a complete body scan known as a 'Computed Axial Tomography' or CAT scan, which provides doctors with a 3D image of the inside of your body, to ensure the cancer was nowhere else. He then said he was also going to book scans to check my bones, bone marrow, breasts and brain. Once they were satisfied that the rest of my body was clear, they could decide how much chemotherapy I would need, and also which type would be most effective in getting rid of all the cancerous cells including any tiny cells too small to be detected by the scans, and if I'd need any radiotherapy after the chemotherapy. He told me to expect the tests to take place within the week, and to start my treatment within the next two weeks. All I could think about was my exams. I had worked so hard, *too* hard, to simply give up half way through. I had proven my GP and the consultant at Queen Mary's wrong, and I had shown my friends and the teachers who had also doubted me that I wasn't simply trying to draw attention to myself. I wanted to do my exams, I wasn't trying to get out of them, I wanted to be successful. So I explained that I was right in the middle of my GCSEs and had another three weeks of exams, plus a highly anticipated party to throw, before any of this could take place. I told him that it would all have to wait. He laughed, admiring my determination and explained that I would need the scans done as soon as possible. But he compromised saying dependant on the results, I may be able to put off the chemotherapy for a few weeks. I wrote down my exam schedule and he took it, promising to try to arrange the scans around them. He then stood up, shook my hand, said he'd be in touch, and left.

I turned to the nurse as she began to explain a little bit about chemotherapy, but I couldn't hear her. The only thing I knew about chemotherapy, from the little I had read and seen from documentaries on TV was that I would lose my hair. I had an image of a small, bald girl, curled up on a hospital bed, attached to a drip, fear and helplessness in her eyes. That's going to be me I thought, I'm going to lose my hair, I could feel my heart thundering in my chest. I had always had a love / hate relationship with my hair. It was a deep auburn, and it always reminded me of my Irish roots. The whole of my grandad's side of the family had red hair, and I was always considered one of them, a true Bennett. But along with that came the bullying in and out of school. The teasing for being ginger and made to feel different and ugly. Now I was faced with losing it I wish I had told all those who had picked on me to fuck off. I wish I'd had the strength to see that I was beautiful, even if I was 'ginger'. In a split second I regretted each and every time I had wished I was brunette, or blonde. If only I could keep my hair through the treatment I would now appreciate it so much more. But the nurse told me it was almost certain that it would fall out. "The treatment you need is too strong for it not to cause hair loss", she explained. She went on to describe how the chemo gets rid of the cancer cells by killing off all cells—good and bad, this is why your hair falls out. She explained the hair on my head as well as that all over my body would fall out, including my eyelashes and eyebrows. Well, I thought, at least I won't have to wax for a while I guess.

Of all the problems and obstacles I was told to expect, losing my hair was the hardest to come to terms with. As a

31

16 year old girl, I just felt absolute despair. What was Pete going to say? How am I going to be able to go out in public ever again? How long will it take to grow back? So many questions were spinning around and around in my mind. My brain was buzzing, a million thoughts filled my head, but I couldn't organise them enough to ask any educated questions just yet. So we left.

The journey home was quiet. My nan's eyes were red; I couldn't stand to see her upset. It sounds mad, but I tried to make her laugh as we sat on the train, joking about anything I could think of. But she just looked at me with such sadness in her eyes, she looked so helpless. I gave her a hug, and told her everything would be fine, this would all go away soon. But of course, in reality I had no idea. I was absolutely terrified.

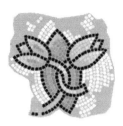

I still had exams to sit; the next one was due to take place in a couple of days. As we reached Sidcup station, grandad was waiting there in the car. Before we pulled away mum told him what the doctor had said. He couldn't believe it, and just sat behind the wheel saying nothing. He drove us home in silence, and as soon as we got in, mum made us all a cup of tea, while we all tried to take everything in. She suggested we go straight to my school to explain the situation to Mrs Hutchinson, my head teacher, as soon as possible. Everything was still so surreal, I agreed and almost in a dream-like state we drank our tea before grandad drove us there. Mum phoned ahead while we were in the car to arrange an immediate meeting with the head teacher.

Outside my school I stepped out of the car, and reality suddenly started hitting hard. I walked past the examination hall, and could see through the windows from the outside the row upon row of students silently setting up their futures. I spotted some of my friends sitting their Home Economics exam, and as I peered through the glass I felt for the first time the barrier between them and me that was set to remain for the next six months. I followed mum and grandad into the entrance hall where we waited to be called by Mrs Hutchinson. She greeted us with a smile, but it soon faded as she saw the three of us struggling to reciprocate her gesture. She shook mum's hand, and invited us into her office. As we followed her down the corridor to her room, she called back to me, "I hope you're ready for Biology on Friday, Natasha", I gave a nervous laugh.

"Yes, Miss", I replied, "of course".

As we walked into her office, she offered us cups of tea and we automatically accepted and sat down around a small table in the centre of the room. "I have to be honest", she said laughing as she re-entered the room having put the kettle on in the small kitchenette next to her office, "I'm a little worried about what you have to say, it must be serious if your grandad's here too!" I let mum do all the talking, I just sat staring at the floor as once again, I heard the words 'cancer', 'chemo' and 'treatment' circling around me. I looked up at my head teacher as she sat in front of me in complete shock. "Goodness me," she stammered, "all those lunch times in the medical room, all those pain killers the hospital sent you home with, all those times they sent you away, I can't believe it, I just can't believe it".

"I want to finish my exams", were the only words I said to her that day.

"Of course you can, but if you want to postpone them, or you need extra time in the examination hall, or you just don't feel like coming in for them one day, you tell me, we'll sort it out, it's no problem. I just can't believe this", she said shaking her head.

We drank our tea as mum explained that we were still a little unsure about what happens next. She told her that I would need scans to see if the cancer had spread anywhere else in my body before they could decide how much chemo and further treatment I would need.

As we got up to leave, Mrs Hutchinson walked over to me and threw her arms around me. I was a little bit taken back! "Er, thanks Miss", I stammered not sure whether it was entirely appropriate to hug her back, but she squeezed me so tight.

"You are going to be fine, do you hear me? Now hurry up and get better, you've got A levels to do too, ok?" I laughed and mum thanked her as we slowly walked back up the corridor towards the main door. "See you Friday then", she said, "don't be late!"

I decided not to tell my friends until after we had sat all of our exams. I didn't want to upset them, and distract them from their studies. I thought they would be devastated for me, and would want to spend some time together to take my mind off what was going to happen. But I wanted them to do well, I wanted them to get on with their revision, and when we saw each other at exam time talk about normal things and not how my last scans went. I also decided not to tell Pete until his exams were over too, he was sitting his AS levels, and there was no way I could drop this on him, I wanted him to do well so I kept it to myself for a while.

It was hard, there were times before my exams when I would overhear people panicking and being over dramatic, saying if they failed these exams their life would be over, their parents would kick them out, they'd never get a good job. Get a fucking grip, I would think to myself looking at them. Walking into school I'd see some girls chain-smoking outside the main entrance, "I'm so nervous, I can't stop shaking", I heard one girl say to her friend as I walked past her while she was lighting up another fag. I felt so angry watching them, living their life, being normal, being teenagers. I couldn't help but feel sorry for myself, no matter how hard I tried to snap myself out of thinking about what I was about to go through, I was frightened, and felt so lonely. It'll be better, I thought to myself, when I tell the girls and Pete, I'll have so much love and support, I just need to get these exams out of the way, things will be so much better when I have my friends around me. I couldn't have been more wrong.

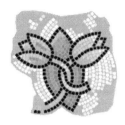

As promised, my consultant arranged the scans around my exams. Every time I had a day free of exams, mum, myself and often grandad would travel back to the Royal Marsden in South Kensington for a day spent in waiting rooms and treatment rooms. I was directed from one department to another for more CAT scans, Magnetic Resonance Imaging Scans (or MRIs), bone scans, breast scans; I had swab samples taken from my nose, ears and all sorts of other places. I felt like a rag doll being pushed and pulled from doctor to radiographer, from radiographer to nurse, all the while I was in a complete daze, still convinced I was stuck in a nightmare I couldn't wake myself up from. I remember being examined by one doctor, he was young, with dark hair, dark eyes and tanned olive skin, he was absolutely gorgeous. He wanted to take my blood pressure, check my breathing and other statistics before I had one of the scans. He told me to lie back on the bed in his tiny office, as he drew the curtains around the bed. He then put his stethoscope in his ears and took the other end in his hand before placing it on my chest underneath my top. I was only young, and was absolutely mortified to have this handsome doctor's hand up my top, my heart started to really pound, "You need to relax", he kept saying getting really impatient with me.

"You've got your hand up my top", I snapped back,

"Just try to relax, yes?" He may have been good-looking, but he had no idea how to talk to a patient, especially a young female, and he didn't exactly make the shitty situation I had been forced into any better for me.

On the day of my final scans I was absolutely exhausted. My first was a breast scan, I felt utterly exposed as the radiographer asked me to undress. I asked if my mum could be with me. She said, "Of course", so mum stood back as I undressed from the waist up. The radiographer guided me over to the scanning machine and angled my body towards what looked like a medieval torture device, with what appeared to be a clamp on the front of it. I brushed aside the wave of fear that fell over me when I wondered if that was the part of the machine your boob is placed inside in order to scan it. I thought to myself don't be ridiculous, that would just be cruel! But as the radiographer pulled and pushed and squeezed, I realised, to my horror my initial thoughts had been correct. The radiographer spent around 15 minutes getting me and my lady parts at just the right angle; my arms had to be in a particular place, my body also had to be in line, and my boob had to be completely clamped in! I felt a bit sorry for it, trapped between the metal bars of the machine. I looked down at my poor squashed boob, convinced it would be forevermore disfigured.

"Ok!" the radiographer said after a while. By this I thought she meant 'ok, you're all done, I can release your boob and off you go'. So I stepped back and relaxed my arms. I was unable to walk away completely, as a certain part of my body was still firmly attached to the machine. Unfortunately, what she actually meant was 'ok, get ready for the scan to start'! So back she came, to put me in place again, pushing and pulling and tugging my body. By now she was understandably a little impatient with me. She was so rough with my body trying to get me back into position quickly, I wondered if she realised that my boob was in fact attached to me, and that I would very much like to take it with me, still attached, when I went home!

When I had completed all the examinations, (still a little sore from boobgate), my designated nurse came to check on me, to make sure that I was ok and that I knew what the next step would be. She asked if I would like to see the ward on which I was due to start treatment the following week, and I agreed. I thought I might as well be prepared for what was waiting for me, so we followed the nurse through a maze of corridors and staircases. As we approached the ward my stomach turned. There was an awful smell in the air that was getting stronger; a combination of stale food, mixed with pee and sick. I walked through the double doors and was confronted by a series of bays, each with six beds, which were all occupied by little old ladies. Some were moaning, others were getting sick. Some were crying to themselves, and others had family around them crying constantly over them. I thought to myself there was no way I could stay here while I had my treatment, the depression I would sink into would surely kill me long before the disease did. I looked around one more time, then glanced at my mum, the expression on her face told me she was equally horrified. My grandad stepped forward and politely asked the nurse if it would be possible for me to have my treatment on one of the children's or possibly a 'young peoples' ward. I turned to him and smiled at his suggestion. But the nurse replied that there was no 'young peoples ward', just the children's ward, and it was the hospital's policy to put me on an adult ward as I had already turned 16. I glanced around at where I would have to stay; I had seen enough. I turned to walk back out of the ward. I noticed the ward sister watching us, she must have overheard our conversation, and thank God she did; she approached us, and put her arm around me. My eyes were filling with tears as the reality of what was happening really began to kick in. But I felt comforted as she held me around my waist, and she looked at my mum and asked if we had heard of the Teenage Cancer Trust Charity. We replied no, and she explained that the trust had set up wards in different cities across the UK, which were designed just for teenagers and young adults to be treated on. The sister went on to explain that the nearest hospital with a Teenage Cancer Trust Unit was, what was then called, the Middlesex Hospital in Goodge Street. The Middlesex Hospital has since closed down, it closed in 2005, but was relocated just a little further up Tottenham Court Road very near to Warren Street tube station, and is now called the University College Hospital. She said it would be no problem to have my hospital file sent over there, and for me to have a new consultant and the treatment I needed on one of these specialist wards. The relief I felt was unimaginable. She offered to get the process in motion for me, and suggested I go to the Middlesex immediately to see if I would be more comfortable there instead so we could get things moving as soon as possible. We thanked her and my grandad shook her hand, we left the Marsden and hailed a taxi to take us across London to Goodge Street. When we arrived, we quickly found the Teenage Cancer Trust Unit, and the staff told us that the lovely nurse from the Marsden had phoned ahead, so there was already a nurse and support assistant waiting for us. They then took mum, grandad and I on a little tour around the ward. It was colourful, bright, the nurses were happy, there was a TV and games room. The ward was large with the beds situated around a pool table. What a difference to the smelly, miserable, dark, depressing ward I was due to be treated on only an hour earlier. I smiled as I said I would be much happier here; it had made such a sad day seem a little bit brighter. The ward staff said they would organise a consultant and medical team who would be in touch over the next few days to let me know exactly when my treatment would start. I spoke to a support nurse, who told me all the procedures that were to happen once my school exams were finished. She explained that I would need what was called a Hickman Line, which is a tube that is inserted into a vein in your neck and comes out just beneath your ribcage. It sounded pretty horrific as she was describing it, but she assured me that it was the best way to administer the chemo. Because the drugs I would need were effectively toxins, it is safer for them to attach the chemo drip to a tube that is securely inserted into a main vein. If they are simply injected into the veins in your arms or in the back of your hands, there is the danger that the vein will be missed, and the medication would poison your body. It also made it much easier for hospital staff to take blood; with all the chemo, your veins tend to collapse, and it's often really hard to carry out even simple blood tests. With a Hickman Line, it's quick, easy and painless to extract blood; you can even learn to do it yourself, as I did much later! As the nurse described the procedure, she also explained that my chemo cycles would last around five days each. I would remain in hospital for the five days, then rest at home for two weeks, until it was time for the next cycle of treatment, which would last another five days. This would continue until the consultants were satisfied that there was either an improvement in my condition, or that perhaps it would be more appropriate to try something else if the disease wasn't clearing. She explained things slowly and clearly; she made sure I understood what she was saying and encouraged me to ask any questions no matter how trivial I thought they might be. As I was listening, I turned to my grandad who was sitting beside me, he had suddenly fallen very silent. He was the type of man who would crack jokes and make you smile even in the most desperate of situations. I remember being with him when one of his sisters was dying; as the head of the entire family it fell to him to keep us all together, and he did this always through humour. We were all so sad standing around her hospital bed but he always managed to bring a little bit of sunshine into the room with his sharp wit and funny stories. But as I turned to look at him now the tears just rolled down his face. "Just get rid of it", he said, "please, get rid of it".

"We'll try", she replied gently.

I had only seen my grandad cry once before, it was Christmas Day 1992, and one of my cousin and I went to visit him in hospital after he had had a huge, near fatal, heart attack. The whole family was crowded around the bed as his two eldest grandchildren were brought into the bay to see him, and as we stood beside the bed holding his hand, his eyes glistened. I was only seven at the time, but I'll never forget the fear and helplessness in his eyes as he lay in the bed, with an oxygen mask over his mouth. The same look was etched on his face now as we sat together in the TV room; there were no jokes, there was no laughing. As the discussion came to a close, a nurse appeared with a date on which I would need to return to have my Hickman Line inserted. It was only a couple of weeks away.

Not long after my induction into the Middlesex, I learned that my scans showed a tiny amount of spotting on my lungs. For me, it justified the need for chemotherapy. Although the rest of my body looked clear on the scans, the chemo would help eradicate these tiny tumours on my lungs, as well as any undetected cancerous cells elsewhere. I was also told I may need radiotherapy on my lungs once the chemo was over, but a decision on that would be made much later when the effects of the chemo became clear.

So that was it, there was nothing left to say. I had two short weeks to enjoy myself, to try to squeeze in as many things that I would miss out on over the next six months. Such a short time in which to celebrate the end of my exams, the freedom of the summer, the excitement of having no studies. In no time at all it would be cruelly snatched away from me in exchange for months in a hospital bed with just a small window to watch the summer pass by.

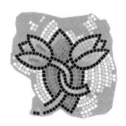

Each year as we were growing up, grandad took the family for a two-week break to Butlins in Minehead, Somerset. They were undoubtedly the best two weeks of the year, and we looked forward to going so much. A few times, my cousins came with my aunt and uncle, but mostly it would just be nan, grandad, mum, Dom and me. As we got older, we stopped renting apartments inside Butlins, and instead would rent a cottage or apartment just outside the camp on the sea front, and it was here that my grandad taught me to drive. It was so important to him that we all learnt how to drive, he knew it was our passport to independence, and we couldn't have asked for a better teacher. I was probably about 14 the first time we took the car to a car park just by the seafront arcade, it was completely empty, and just beside it was a fabulous sort of makeshift bike track with hills and bumps and all sorts. Grandad drove Dominic, Dominic's bike and myself to the car park, and as Dominic cycled around almost breaking his neck over the hills and rubble, grandad taught me to drive. He taught me all the manoeuvres I needed to know, and as we were in a car park, I mastered the art of all sorts of parking, forwards, backwards, sideways, all before I was even 16. I couldn't wait to get my provisional licence and start driving properly on the roads. For a little while, if grandad and I were in the car together he would stop at the end of his road, and let me drive the rest of the way, not entirely legal, but I loved the feeling of driving him around, even if it was for just 30 seconds until we pulled up on his drive!

A couple of weeks after I was diagnosed, grandad told me he had a surprise for me, but it wasn't in the house, we had to pop down the road to pick it up. I was confused, but obviously excited, although not as excited as he was, but what could it be that we had to go and pick it up? I thought maybe it may have been a puppy, but we already had a lovely little dog, maybe it was a dress, and some new shoes, but why would we have to pick them up? Mum came with us, and as we drove up to the high street he kept saying that it's ok if I don't like it, all I have to do is tell him, we can get another one instead. But I was so excited, I just wanted to see what it was, and as we got closer grandad was dying to get out of the car to show me. Just then, we pulled into a second-hand car showroom. I nearly died, I hadn't yet turned 17—the legal age to start learning to drive, but grandad had seen a small plum-coloured metro the day before and had fallen in love with it. As we got out of the car the salesman walked over to us, "Ah, Mr Bennett, lovely to see you again!"

"Yes chief", grandad replied, "we've brought her up to see what she thinks". I thought it was perfect. Grandad left the salesman to show me the interior of the car, and walked around the showroom looking at what else was on offer. I was so excited as I got into the driver's seat, just as grandad strolled back towards us saying, "Now if you don't like it, just say, you've got plenty of time to get another one".

"I love it grandad, but you're right, I do have a lot of time. Let me get my treatment over with, then I can get a job and put money towards it with you".

"Natasha, if you like it, we'll get it. It's a good price, and you'll be able to practice off-road in the evenings". I didn't know what to say. My lovely grandad was buying me a car. My own car all to myself, what could I say to that?

"Thank you grandad, I would like it very much".

"Where do I sign?" he said to the salesman. So that was that, he put the car in my name, signed a cheque, and mum and I jumped in and mum drove it home.

He couldn't make me better, he couldn't take the disease away, he couldn't have the treatment for me, I knew he would if he could, so I guess this was the one thing he could do for me to make me feel a little better. My little metro and I were inseparable from that day on, I kept her clean, kitted her out with a pink, fluffy interior, much to grandad's dismay, and once I had passed my test, drove her everywhere. I can see now that along with the car, grandad gave me the best present I could ever ask for, independence and freedom; a gift, after months spent in hospital, I would soon learn to treasure.

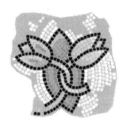

The day of my last exam soon arrived. It was another English exam, which was perfect as all my friends were there and so I decided to tell them about my treatment when it was over. Before we went into the examination hall, I asked them all not to rush off as soon as we were allowed to leave, as I had something to tell them. They all got really excited and wanted me to tell them there and then. I laughed, and said, "No, believe me it can wait, let's get this out of the way first". They thought it might have something to do with the party I had organised which was finally taking place the following Friday night, a surprise guest maybe. We were soon ushered into the hall in silence, and as the exam began, I started to really panic. I realised that as soon as this was over my treatment would start. While the exams had been going on I always had something between me and the chemo, I had something else to get out of the way first, I had a distraction and something to focus on, now there was nothing. The English exam we were sitting was a creative writing test, and the question asked us to write about our idea of the perfect island. I wrote about freedom,

I thought about being as far away from Sidcup and chemo, and treatment and cancer as I could. I wrote about being free to breathe on a perfect, untouched beach surrounded by nature and the sound of the sea lapping the shore. I described a feeling of exhilaration at just being me, of having no one to account to, no responsibilities, no regrets and no fears. I wrote and wrote until I was told to put my pen down, and as the examination hall was cleared row by row, I thought about how desperately I wanted to be on that island.

"So". Lucy said, unable to contain herself, "What's this exciting news?" The girls stood around me in a crowd expectantly.

"Er, Lucy, I didn't say it was exciting! Anyway, remember all those stomach pains I had months ago, when I couldn't move and spent every lunch hour in the medical room?"

"Oh, yeah", they replied.

"Well, a couple of weeks ago I had to go back to the hospital, they did a biopsy on the mass of cells they found, and I got the results. It's cancer".

"What?" Lucy asked as she let out a little impulse laugh, "are you kidding?" The others just stood there, and I saw a tear roll down one of their faces.

"No, I'm not joking, why would I joke about something like this?"

"You're still going to have your party though?" was Lucy's next question. I should have known from the concern she showed that day the amount of support I could expect from my best friend, and I just stood looking at her as she had caught me completely off guard.

"Er, yes I'm still having the party, God knows I need it after the two months I've just had", I carried on, "then next week I have to go into hospital for what's known as a Hickman Line to be inserted". I explained to them what that was, then told them the doctors had told me what treatment I would need, I said that I wouldn't be in school much, but I was going to try so hard not to let it affect my studies and I'd be back again all fixed before I knew it. I was trying to convince myself I think, rather than any of my friends, who just stood there looking at me not really sure of what to say. But I could understand this. At that age I doubt I'd have had any idea what I should say if it had been the other way around, and one of them was telling me that they had this terrifying disease, with no idea whether they would survive it. So I told them all not to worry, not to be sad, and we'd have a great time on Friday. And we did. The party was held in a local church hall, mum splashed out on a cheesy DJ, and nan and grandad organised the balloons and decorations for inside the hall. I spent all day getting ready, I had my nails done, I curled my hair, threw on a new outfit and heels and I danced all night. I danced to forget what waited for me on the other side of the weekend, I danced for all the nights I would be stuck in hospital when I should have been out with my friends, I danced until the last person had left and mum took me home, exhausted.

The next day, I wondered if I should call Pete, but quickly thought better of it. I had spoken to him a few days before on the evening of his last exam. We spoke about going on a date—our first one since we decided to cool things down before my GCSEs. I told him how much I had missed him and couldn't wait to see him, but that things might be a little difficult for a while. Then I explained what had caused my bad stomach pains. I had hidden the pain from him as much as I could, I was embarrassed about having bad period pains or whatever it had been diagnosed as that week, and not being able to eat in front of him.

I never really complained too much to him, and it wasn't until I had the operation that I explained just how much pain I had been in. I went on to describe what was to come, and how ill I was going to be. I told him I wanted to see him as much as I could, and mum could take me over to his house, and she would pick him up and bring him round to ours, but as I was talking I could tell he was freaking out. After a long pause he asked, "Will your hair fall out?"

"Probably", I said as my heart gave a great thud.

"Shit." He fell silent again. "Oh, mum's calling me for dinner, I'll ring you back after I've eaten, ok?"

"Yeah, fine", I replied, "don't rush your food, I'll be in the rest of the afternoon". But he didn't call back; in fact he never called again. I could understand how unsure he must have been, frightened himself perhaps, afraid of what his mates would say if he was seen with a bald girl, but I was broken. My world was collapsing on top of me, and when I turned to him for support he showed how much of a coward he was. I saw him again, quite recently actually, I was with mum and grandad in a supermarket, and he looked me straight in the eye before diving behind one of the aisles. I laughed as I thought how spineless he was, after all these years he was still running away! As if we hadn't all moved on! People like that will always be running I guess, running from their past, running from their fears, never able to look terror in the eye and face things head on. As I was leaving the store, I saw him pay for his shopping and I watched as he stroked his girlfriend's hair, much like how you would stroke a dog, what a lucky escape that was I thought as I smiled to myself, and walked out of the shop.

"But he that dares not grasp the thorn,
should never crave the Rose"

Anne Bronte

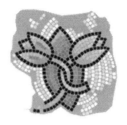

I had no idea what to expect the day I walked onto that ward in the Middlesex Hospital for my Hickman Line to be inserted. I had been told to get there for around nine in the morning, and as I entered breakfast was just being wheeled out. It was funny, I had been there looking around the ward only a few weeks previously, yet I hardly remembered it at all. I had barely taken in any of the real detail about the ward, the décor, the atmosphere, the people. There were seven beds in the main part of the ward, and several side rooms. There was a large bathroom at one end of the ward, and at the other there was a small games and TV room, with a tiny toilet opposite. Next to the loo was the kitchen, where you were able to store and prepare your own food if you weren't too keen on the hospital food. There was artwork all around the walls along with photos of the patients; for a ward treating young patients with cancer, it was so welcoming and vibrant. I was introduced to a couple of the nurses before the doctors began their ward rounds, and in the meantime I unpacked my little case and tried to settle in. But all the other patients looked so ill, I felt almost frightened to go up to each of them and introduce myself, so instead I sat on my bed and smiled over at them. They looked back at me with their bald heads, and dark sunken eyes. Some of their faces looked so empty, so expressionless as they each lifted a hand to gesture back at me. Surrounded by drips, dialysis machines and other equipment I didn't recognise, my heart sunk as the reality of this next stage of my life smacked me straight in the face. "This is going to be me in a few weeks", I whispered to mum. "I can't tell which patients are girls, and which are boys", I said desperately and my eyes filled with tears as she looked back at me, unable to say anything that would comfort me. A nurse came over, and sat on my bed next to me. She had a few forms for me to fill out, she wanted to know if I smoked or drank, how tall I was, how much I weighed. I wanted to run away, get up and walk out of there, I didn't want to look like the people in the beds around me. As I looked around I thought no, I don't smoke, and I don't drink, in fact I really look after myself, so why the hell was this happening to me?

That day I was also introduced to my new consultant, Dr Jeremy Whelan. He came into the ward and sat next to me on my bed, so calm, very reassuring, and so refreshingly honest. He is probably the only doctor to have been completely straight with me throughout all of my treatment, no matter what the news or how much he knows I don't want to hear it, he always tells me how it is. His honesty makes me feel safe, I know that he's not withholding any information from me to make me feel better, or to soften the blow. He gives me the complete picture, and so now I often have great difficulty having consultations with anyone else, even his most trusted registrars. He had with him the results from all the scans I had had done at the Royal Marsden in a large file which he placed next to him on the mattress.

"Do I really need all this?" I asked him, "I've had my operation, can I not just come back for scans every now and then, to make sure it isn't causing too much damage? What will happen if I don't have this chemo?"

"You'll die, Natasha. The rest of your scans show you have spotting on your lungs, and there may well be other minute cancerous cells throughout your body that aren't detectable on our scans. These tiny spots on your lungs will grow, and at some point, sooner or later it will kill you. It's your choice". Harsh, but at least I knew where I stood, and now I knew for sure that, of course, I had no choice.

"Ok".

He then told me I needed to sign the consent form for the Hickman Line operation. He explained again the benefits of having it inserted, how much easier it would be to administer the chemo, and take blood, how much more hygienic it would be but his words washed over me as I read the warnings and dangers of the operation on the form. He explained that looking at my scans, they would need to administer six cycles of chemo for now, one cycle would take around five days, with a two week break before I would need to come back for the next one. When the six cycles were over, they would rescan my whole body, and make a decision about any further treatment I might need. I picked up the pen the consultant had placed next to me on the bed and as I scanned the page, "Death by piercing of the heart" stopped me from putting pen to paper, I could feel my blood turning cold.

"What the fuck is this?" I said, pointing to the sentence.

"Well, the tube is inserted very near to the heart, Natasha, there's only a very small chance it could happen, but it is something we have to make you aware of. Look, the benefits to having this procedure are immeasurable, and the dangers of having the chemo fed through a line in your arm are equally as substantial as those in front of you now. I can't tell you what to do, but I can advise you, and I advise you that this is your best option. So I signed it. Having turned 16 a few weeks before, I was no longer legally considered a child so was now old enough to give my consent to any operations and procedures I had from now on. Mum always says how difficult she finds it watching me sign form after form for operations, chemo, and other treatments I've had over the years.

"You're my baby" she always says, "I should be able to take this away from you", but there was nothing she could do for me now as I signed and dated the bottom of the Hickman Line form and handed it back to Dr Whelan.

I woke up a couple of hours later, and cried out. As I tried to open my eyes, everything was really blurry. The light shone so brightly in my face, I couldn't move or speak, I just wanted my mum. A nurse came rushing over and stroked my forehead. "Well done chick", she reassured me, "it's all over now, you're in recovery, so we'll fetch mum, then you can go back up to the ward and rest some more". I tried to nod as I closed my eyes, relieved that it was all over, and I was alive. I woke up properly a few hours later. Mum was by my bed and nan and grandad had come up with Dominic while I was sleeping. "How are you feeling honey? Can you sit up?" As I tried to pull myself up, I yelped in pain. I was in absolute agony all the way down my left side, it took my breath away.

"No!" I squealed as I gently lowered myself back onto the mattress. A nurse came over to take my blood pressure, "Can I have some painkillers please?" I asked her.

"Of course you can! I'll get you some now". Once she was happy with my blood pressure reading, she walked over to the medication cabinet which was nailed to a wall behind the nurse's desk. She came back to the bed with two paracetamol tablets in a small cup and a glass of water accompanied by a straw. She broke the pills in half for me and I swallowed them as I slurped some water from the cup. "For the moment just try to stay as still as you can, if you need to use the loo, give us a shout we'll bring over the commode to you".

"How long is this going to last? The pain is incredible!"

"It will start to ease off soon, you'll be hurting for a couple of days, and you'll just be uncomfortable for a few days after that. This time next week you'll be up and about as normal".

"Ok thanks, that doesn't seem so bad I guess", I said, looking at mum feeling a little relieved. But she was wrong; I was in agony for the following two weeks. I was so frightened and confused, and I was angry that I had been told to expect to be 'uncomfortable', when in reality, I could hardly breathe the pain was so intense. And so began my frustration with the hospital staff for sugar coating the information they gave me. Telling me that things would be a lot better and less painful than they actually were made me feel reassured at the time, but in the long run left me scared and anxious.

The day after the operation, the hospital discharged me, saying I would be more comfortable recovering at home. I was in absolute agony as grandad picked mum and I up from the Middlesex and took us home. I tried to stretch out on the back seat as much as I could, as if I was lying on a bed, but I just couldn't get comfortable, I couldn't wait to get home to be able to relax properly for a couple of days until hopefully the pain began to subside. The hospital instructed me to call them and let them know when I was feeling better so they could arrange a bed for me and I could get my chemo started. I assumed this would be at the beginning of the following week at the very latest from what the nursing staff had told me, but I was in pain for much longer than I was told to expect, and the wait was terrifying.

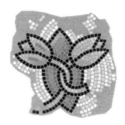

I realise that for some people it is easier to deal with the treatment and side effects if the information they are offered was in some way filtered, with some aspects of the reality of what was about to happen perhaps missing or at least glossed over. I guess it softened the blow, made things a little less terrifying, or daunting. But I didn't feel like that, and neither did many of the other teenagers I spoke to about it on the ward. Indeed, treating people with cancer at such a sensitive age, I have seen, presents a tricky situation to many inexperienced medical staff. Firstly, they are often unsure of who even to speak to, you or your parents. I found it so infuriating when a young doctor would talk over my head and tell my mum about the treatment I was to have. So much so, that often I would be cheeky and break the conversation asking mum if I was invisible? She would just laugh and throw me a look that told me to behave myself, as the doctor shifted uncomfortably but then directed their speech at me instead. "Please talk to *me*", I would say, "*I* am your patient, *I* am having the treatment, *I* would like to know how *I'm* going to feel. Please, don't ignore me".

However, on the other hand when I was being spoken to, I often found that a lot of the information was held back. On many occasions after I had had an operation, such as my Hickman Line being inserted, or some treatment, or a procedure had been carried out I was told to expect to feel uncomfortable for perhaps a few days, or weeks, but the reality was very different. After my Hickman had been fitted I lay in bed unable to move, eat or go to the toilet for the next two weeks. I worried that something must have been very wrong, and I would call the ward nearly every other day telling them that I was still hurting, that something unexpected must have happened during the operation. After a week of lying in bed holding my side, I remember thinking in a panic, what if they have left some sort of surgical instrument inside me?! I couldn't understand why I was still in so much pain when I should have only been "uncomfortable" for five days at the very most. After two weeks of calling the hospital and getting no reassuring answers I asked to speak to my consultant, Dr Whelan. I was transferred to his office, by which time I was a little hysterical telling him that something had definitely gone wrong, and I was coming back to the hospital in the morning. But in his usual calm soothing tone, he simply replied, "Please don't panic Natasha, everything is fine, in fact you may indeed still be in the same amount of pain this time next week. You've had a very invasive procedure, and your body needs time to heal. Give yourself time to rest and recover." I put the phone down and wondered why the nurses hadn't told me this the first time I called them more than a week previously. If I had been told as soon as I came round from the operation, 'look love, you'll be in agony for weeks, and unable to go to the toilet independently for a month' I wouldn't have been thrilled about it, but at least I would have been prepared. I wouldn't have been panicking every morning when I woke up and the pain was still as sharp as when I went to sleep. I wouldn't be worried about a scalpel being left inside me, or having some sort of hideous infection. I would have known that although my body was taking its time to heal, at least it *was* healing.

Much later on during my treatment, after one of my cycles I was leaving the ward and I noticed in one of the side rooms a girl around the same age as me. She was standing by her windowsill, putting up all her 'get well soon' cards and balloons, and, like the rest of us, trying to make her new little living space as comfortable and homely as possible. As I walked past her I smiled, and her mum appeared from behind the door. My mum nodded hello to her as she stepped out of the room towards us. "Are you all finished then?" she asked positively.

"For now", mum replied, "we have a few more cycles before they let us go for good!"

The girl introduced herself. "I'm Amanda" she said, "I'm in for my first treatment soon, but tomorrow I have the operation to put my Hickman Line in"

"How do you feel about it?" I asked.

"Ok", she replied, "they said I'll be uncomfortable for a few days, then after that I'll be right as rain, and back to normal!" I couldn't believe it! She had been told exactly the same thing as me, obviously to make her feel more relaxed about what was coming. But I couldn't let her go through the confusion, anxiety and worry that I went through when my Hickman Line was inserted. I told her to expect to be much more than 'uncomfortable', and that the pain was more likely to last two weeks, rather than just two days. I explained that obviously everybody has different and very individual experiences, but generally it was very likely to be more painful and for a much longer time than had been suggested to her. She thanked me, and although I'm sure this new information had made her a little more concerned she said she preferred not to have the information sugar coated. Like me, and many others on the ward, she wanted to know what was to come, and be ready for it.

Having the Hickman Line was the best decision I made. My chemo was fed through so easily, it was safe, quick and hygienic and I learned to take blood through it myself. In between cycles, I had to take blood samples and deliver them to my local hospital Queen Mary's, they would relay the results to the Middlesex in London so that they could keep an eye on me, and make sure there were no nasty infections lurking ready to cause havoc in my body! I was given tiny blood tubes, syringes, flushes and wipes, as well as a special hygiene bin to dispose of them in, known as a 'sharpsbin'. It was the one tiny bit of independence I was able to hold on to throughout the whole nightmare, taking care of my Hickman Line, flushing it to keep it clean and clear and taking blood for the hospital. When the hospital received the blood I had taken, they would carry out tests on it which would show them if my kidneys were malfunctioning, or if there was a problem with my liver, or other organs. At first the nurses at the Middlesex and Queen Mary's did all the work for me, but after a couple of months I learned to do it myself. It was quite simple extracting the blood from my Hickman Line and distributing it in the little tubes I was provided with, but it made me feel useful, it made me feel that I could rely on myself to look after myself, I didn't always need a medic running round after me. For the first time in a long time I felt very proud of myself.

The line caused me no problems at all, and I was told to wrap it up onto my skin and stick it to myself with a plaster.

But I always seemed to suffer a reaction to the plasters they gave me, they made my skin red and itchy, I couldn't keep them on any longer than two minutes! So I tucked the line into my trousers to keep it from hanging down and pulling on my skin with the elastic. The hospital staff would go crazy when they saw it tucked into my clothes and not kept up and out of the way with a plaster, but it didn't matter because that's what worked for me, the line caused me no problems and it never got infected, it was literally my lifeline.

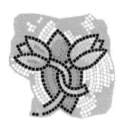

As the pain of the Hickman Line eventually began to subside, I thought about calling the hospital to arrange going back in to start my treatment. What if I don't call them? I thought to myself, I don't have to go back there, I don't have to go through this. But Dr Whelan's words rang in my ears, "It's your choice" echoed in my mind over and over again. So I picked up the phone and dialled the number to the ward, they told me if I was ready I could come in early the following morning, as they had a spare bed. I thought about it for a while, deliberating whether I should give myself another week of freedom, but I knew I'd always just want another week, and another week, so I decided it was probably better to get on with it. "Well" I said to the nurse, "I guess the sooner I start it, the sooner it will be over".

"Exactly", she replied, and I put the phone down.

"Tomorrow", I said to mum who was listening as she sat on the sofa with a cup of tea.

"Ok", she said, "ok", and we cuddled in front of the TV for the rest of the evening.

I didn't sleep much that night, so I got up early and packed a bag for the week, I brought with me a few home comforts, photographs, my favourite slippers and a little teddy. I felt like a little girl again, I was so terrified. A few hours later as I sat on the hospital bed clutching the cuddly toy my fear turned once again to anger, I just wanted to be normal, to go out with my mates, to have fun. I didn't have too much time to feel sorry for myself though, a doctor surrounded by students walked onto the ward, spoke to a nurse briefly, picked up a huge file and walked over to my bed. She was young with lovely long, curly, blonde hair. I kept staring at it thinking how lucky she was that it wasn't all about to fall out. She introduced herself, and shook my mum's hand. It was only a brief visit, she explained that I would need a chest X-ray, before I started my chemo later that evening. I asked why it was going to take so long, and she replied by saying that the chemo had to sit in the fridge for a few hours, before it could be administrated. Also, the chemo often makes you really tired, so it just makes sense for the chemo to be fed for 12 hours at night when your body is used to sleeping. She went on to explain in more detail what would happen over the coming week, and I learned that the chemo would be administered over five days. The medication would be fed through the night, but during the day, saline would be fed through my Hickman Line in order to clean it out, and rehydrate my body ready for the next dose of chemo the following night. At the end of the five days, I would be able to go home and relax until it was time to come back to the Middlesex two weeks later for another cycle, which would again last five days. This would continue until I'd had six cycles, and then the doctors could review my scans and see what follow up treatment, if any, was needed.

She suggested I go out after the X-ray and have a look around the shops before I was tied to the bed for the next week. Once she left, a nurse came straight over to let me know the X-ray department was ready for me. The nurse took my phone number so she could let me know when I needed to come back to start my treatment and I picked up my handbag and mum and I left. After my X-ray, we walked up and down Oxford Street in silence, we walked in and out of shops, picking things up, then putting them back down. My mind wasn't on shopping at all. All the time I was waiting for my phone to ring, calling me back for the nightmare to begin. It was strange waiting for the call, the time seemed to drag, but at the same time, I wanted that day to last forever, I didn't want to go back to that ward. After a while, having still not heard from the hospital, mum and I found a little coffee shop. We sat and ordered a drink, and a small cake each, and as I picked around the edges of it, I thought about the other patients we had met that day. I thought about the reality that some young people faced of ending their days there, and the reality that I might end my days there. Mum asked me what I was thinking, "Nothing really", I replied, sighing as I lifted my coffee cup to drink from it. Just then my phone rang, I was so startled I nearly dropped the cup. I answered it, and a voice at the other end simply said, "Natasha? We're ready now". My heart began to pound and my hands were really shaking as I gathered my things together. Mum left some change on the table and we walked the small distance back to the hospital. Walking through the main doors squeezing past all the smokers sitting outside I remember feeling so angry. If this could happen to me, someone who was young and otherwise healthy, who didn't smoke, drink, or take drugs, what were these silly people standing here puffing away doing? Why weren't they helping themselves? Some of them were very obviously on treatment, with their bald heads, and their drips attached to their arms. Others were in wheelchairs, with a leg missing, or only one arm, I felt like screaming at all of them, 'Stop killing yourselves!' But instead, I held my breath and walked through the thick cloud of smoke into the building. Mum held my hand all the way back up to the ward, and as we entered, I saw my chemo drip ready and waiting for me next to my bed. It was a large bag of fluid, much like a saline feed, but with another bag over the top of it. The cover was black and yellow, and had the word 'TOXIC' written all over it. A nurse came over to me smiling, and asked how I was feeling, I said nothing back to her as she put on her gloves, opened an 'alcho-wipe', which was a hygiene wipe and cleaned the ends of my Hickman Line. I watched as she attached the bottom of the drip to my Hickman, and then opened the top of the drip to allow the fluid to begin slowly feeding through. The nurse then advised me to get ready for bed, so that if I started to feel sick or tired, I could just fall asleep comfortably. Before I got changed though, she quickly mentioned that every time I needed to use the loo, I should use the jugs found in the bathroom, then she turned and went to leave. "Excuse me?" I shouted, "you want me to pee in a jug?"

"Yes, we need to monitor how much fluid is going in, but also, how much is coming out".

"Er, well can't I just tell you when I go?" I asked in disgust.

"No, we need to monitor exactly how much is coming out, and the content".

"Ok, fine", I replied, completely deflated.

I lay back on the bed and slowly watched the fluid drip down through the long tube and into my Hickman Line, and as I lay there mum rubbed my forehead. She asked me if I was hungry, or whether I would like a drink, but I shook my head as I started to feel more and more tired. I fell asleep as she stroked my hair, hoping I'd wake up in the morning and the first lot would be over. I opened my eyes after what felt hours, but the lights in the ward were still on. I was blinded as I looked around to see many visitors still sitting around the other beds in the ward. I looked at the clock, I'd only been asleep for half an hour! Suddenly I had a huge urge to use the loo. I jumped up and ran, wincing in pain. I completely forgot I was attached to the drip and as I had run around the bed, my Hickman Line pulled at my skin. I yelped and mum jumped up to help me. "Let me come with you", she said, and she put her arm around me and pushed my drip as I walked slowly to the bathroom. I felt groggy and dizzy as I shuffled through the ward, and I could feel my bladder getting fuller and fuller with each step.

"Oh, quick mum!" I said as we bundled into the bathroom. I looked at the toilet, and it was a complete mess. "How am I supposed to use that?" I cried.

"It's fine honey, I'll sort it out, here" mum said as he passed me a jug which she had found on a ledge behind the toilet. I just looked at her. "I'm sorry honey, you have to". I was so desperate, she quickly cleaned the toilet seat and I used the jug over it. As I put the jug back on the ledge I cried. As if all this wasn't undignified enough, I had to pee in a jug and then put it on display. As I looked up I noticed a row of full jugs, each with a paper towel beneath it with a name written on it. There was a paper towel at the end of the row, with 'Natasha' scrawled at the top of it, I placed my half full jug on it. Then the smell hit me. As I walked over to the sink, I noticed there was no window open, the smell became overpowering, and I felt myself fall backwards. The next thing I remember was waking up sitting on a chair by the sink with my mum and a nurse beside me, still in the toilet, still with no window open, and still surrounded by the stench of piss.

"I need to get out of here",

"No, Natasha, stay here and catch your breath for a second", the nurse commanded.

"I can't breathe! That's the problem! I need to get out!" I leapt up from the chair and rushed out of the bathroom onto the ward. From then on I absolutely dreaded using the bathroom. Sitting in the bath trying to wash with the full jugs lined up and the smell lingering, I never felt clean no matter how much I washed myself, that smell followed me everywhere while I was on the ward.

Unfortunately, my relationship with the bathroom did not much improve, over the coming months. Suffice to say, some other patients' bathroom etiquette left something to be desired! I would dread the moment I had a sudden urge to go shuffling to the other side of the ward. It would be a race against time to get up, untangle the drip from the bedclothes, find my slippers, unplug the drip from the wall and waddle over to the bathroom. Once there, who knew what delights awaited me all over the floor and the seat!

One evening my aunt came to visit me, she had brought with her a wash bag and a change of clothes and said that she would like to stay at the hospital overnight. She wanted to give my mum a break, give her a chance to see her friends, sleep in her own bed, and have some time away from the nightmare. After putting up a bit of a fight mum gave in, and she drove my aunt's car home, promising to be back before I woke in the morning. I was so glad she would be getting a break. There was a parents' room on the ward with a bed, but it was sometimes occupied by other patient's family. Most of the mums stayed with their teens while they were in for chemo, so they took it in turns to sleep in a comfortable bed in the side room set aside especially for parents. So mum often had to put up with a night on a hard chair next to my bed. I hoped that she relaxed, and enjoyed a glass of wine in front of the TV knowing that I was safe and being looked after. Although deep down, I knew she would be thinking of me the whole night desperate to get back to the hospital in the morning.

I was drifting off to sleep when once again all the fluid being pumped into me got the better of my bladder. I jumped up and began my routine battle with the drip, and the bedclothes and the wires. My aunt asked if I needed help, and if I wanted her to come with me. I appreciated her kindness and thoughtfulness, but I didn't want her to see me and my jug! "No, no, I'll be ok, thank you!" I exclaimed. I hurriedly shuffled to the toilet, but it was an absolute mess. There was tissue all over the place and the floor was soaking wet. I couldn't go in wearing my pretty pink fluffy slippers, so I turned back and headed for the tiny loo at the other end of the ward opposite the TV room. As I rushed past my aunt, she looked worried and asked if I was ok. "I can't use that one" I called to her as I wheeled my drip past her. I just made it to the other loo, which, by the way, was so tiny I had to leave my drip outside the door! Everybody sitting in the TV room could see me through the little gap, as the door was held open slightly by the wire feeding my medication. Feeling much better, I came back to my bed but my aunt was nowhere to be seen. I sat on the bed and waited, but after about 15 minutes she still hadn't come back. I thought perhaps she had gone downstairs to get some fresh air, or to go to the shop, so I asked the nurse if I could pop downstairs for a while to see if she was ok.

The nurse explained that I wasn't allowed as the medication was so toxic, that if I fell while I was outside the ward, and pulled the drip down with me, the fluid could spill and pose a threat to others in the hospital. I shrugged and said "ok", and walked towards the main doors of the ward to see if she was perhaps on her way back. As I made my way over, I noticed someone moving around in the main bathroom. I turned and looked in and there was my aunt! I stood staring in shock, she was on her hands and knees scrubbing the floor. The toilet roll had all been picked up, the jugs—most of them full, had been lined up neatly, and she was cleaning all the piss off the floor. The tears streamed down my face. I couldn't even bring myself to use the toilet, and here she was on her knees, cleaning the mess someone else had made so the rest of us could feel a little more comfortable.

I soon noticed that I became very sensitive to all the smells around the ward. Dr Whelan had warned me that this might happen. The smell of lunch and dinner in the evenings used to really bother me. I couldn't stand it, the thought of eating anything off the trolley made me feel physically sick, so everyday when lunch arrived at one o clock and then dinner at five o clock, I would routinely close the curtain and bury myself under the covers until I was sure the food had been cleared and the trolley was on its way back down to the kitchen. After a while, I discovered that the only smells I could really cope with were lavender and mint. I remember one day waking up from a long afternoon nap on the ward, and mum had been out to the shops to get some fresh air. She had come back to me with loads of air fresheners in her bag. She knew that the smell of the ward was getting to me, and tried to think of a way to overpower it, and she came up with air fresheners! They were all lavender and they all smelt so good! I arranged two on my pillow and one under the duvet, so that I could close my eyes and pretend I was far away from the hospital. I could pretend I was anywhere, out in a fresh open field surrounded by the smells of nature, and not rigged up to a toxic medication that was stripping away every part of my dignity. I would bring my own pillows and duvet covers too. Many of the other patients would do the same, to remind them of home, to help them feel more comfortable and relaxed. I used to bring mine so I could bury my head in the pillow and breathe in the fresh fabric conditioner. Of course, it reminded me of home too, and for a while I could pretend I was in my own bed, in my own room, in my own house, but most importantly, it blocked out all of the smells on the ward, it covered up the smell of the food, and it smothered the smell of hygiene wipes. Not content with burying myself in air fresheners and pillows, I used to get my poor mum to either chew mint chewing gum, or eat mints all day, because she would be sitting next to me constantly it meant the smell of mint was always around! I remember thinking how lovely it was, it smelt so fresh compared to the stench of piss and food. The poor woman must have spent all her spare change on minty freshness for me, but she did it, and told everyone else in the family, when they came to visit, to do the same!

Having been on the ward now for a couple of days, I realised I had no choice but to try and relax as the medication was feeding through my Hickman. I was given chemo through the night, then saline all throughout the day, to keep the line clear, clean and flushed. It meant I could never leave the ward, made it impossible to change my top, and I always needed the loo! The chemo made me so sleepy throughout the day despite it only being administered at night, and I often drifted in and out of consciousness as mum chatted away to me about the other patients she had met, what was in the paper that day, the gossip she had heard when she popped across the road to the café that morning for a cup of tea. I tried so hard to keep awake to chat back to her, but I just couldn't keep my eyes open, the chemo was completely knocking me out. I'd fall asleep mid-sentence, in between asking for a drink and drinking it, saying I needed to go to the toilet and actually getting up to go. It was like a type of narcolepsy overcame me for those few days I was attached to the chemo drip, but I was grateful, it could have been much worse. There was a girl in the bed next to me that first week I was on the ward, her head was constantly in a bucket. She couldn't eat or drink a thing without bringing it all back up, and despite it being very unpleasant to hear her getting sick all day every day, my heart broke for her every time she tried to eat something but just couldn't keep it down. She looked over at me with such envy in her eyes, "I wish I could just sleep", she would say, "just stop getting sick and sleep" she often sighed as she flopped back onto the bed and the nurse took her bucket away to be cleaned for the umpteenth time that day.

Towards the end of the week, I had a visit from a dietician, she had a chart with her that showed all the important food groups in my diet. I smiled as it reminded me of the home economics classes I used to enjoy just a couple of years previously at school, learning about the importance of a healthy diet, and how to reflect this in your everyday meal preparation. She explained to me that the chemo may affect my taste buds, I may go off certain foods that I normally love, and could very well start eating others I would never have touched before. She also warned mum that I might fancy one type of food one minute, but once it was prepared may have gone off it completely and changed my mind about what I wanted to eat. She stood at the side of the bed as she explained that when I went home in between cycles, I should try as hard as possible to eat a balanced diet everyday. As she was speaking the girl in the bed beside me laughed, "That's a joke isn't it?", she called over, still clinging onto her bucket, and the dietician stopped talking. She looked at her sympathetically, removed her glasses and sat on the bed next to me. She put her papers down.

"Look," she continued in a much less formal tone, "we like you to eat as much of a balanced diet as you can obviously, but sometimes that's not possible" and she looked over at the girl next to me. She carried on, "when you're feeling low and sick eat what you can, and when you start to get better before the next cycle starts if you fancy eating a dirty, fat, greasy burger eat it, you don't know when you're going to feel like eating again". I laughed and thanked her. Before she left, she said she would order some special diet drinks for me. They were a sort of milkshake that were good for when you didn't feel like eating. A bit like a protein shake, they came in many different flavours, they were great for bulking you up a little if you were feeling really sick and hadn't eaten properly for a while, but they were absolutely disgusting! I just couldn't get on with them at all, I tried every flavour twice, and spat them out each time!

"Oh dear", mum teased, "the dietician's not going to be happy with you at all!"

"You drink them! She'll never know!" I joked back. It was a strange feeling when my taste buds started to change. As well as going off foods, I started to really crave other things, like sausage rolls, green peppers with ketchup on them, onion ring crisps, and milk. That's all I would eat all day every day. I went off milk chocolate completely, it tasted very metallic, and no matter how many times I tried to eat it, each time I had to give up and hand the rest of the bar to mum, who promptly gobbled it up! The only chocolate I learned to be able to eat was white chocolate buttons. Mum would buy packets of them, and they were so sweet and tasty when I had finished a packet of them I would run my finger all the way round the inside of the bag mopping up the tiny bits that had escaped first time round.

Soon it was time to go home, I had finished my first cycle of treatment. The five days were up. Mum had packed our bags the evening before and I couldn't wait to get out of there! I couldn't wait to sleep in my own bed, pee into a toilet rather than a jug, and to see my friends again.

I was sitting at the edge of the bed waiting to be released, (I say released rather than discharged, because I had felt like a prisoner all week, tied to that drip), when a nurse came over to explain what the next procedure would be. She explained that I needed to wait for a few items to come up from pharmacy, I would need anti-sickness tablets and mouth-wash amongst other things. She told me to use the mouth-wash daily to avoid infections in my mouth, and to keep my Hickman Line clean. She told mum that she had arranged for a local Macmillan nurse to come round over the next couple of days to see how I was getting on, and she warned her that many mums had described taking their kids away after that first treatment as going home with a new born baby for the first time. She said to take things as they happen, and to call the ward at any time if we had any problems or questions. There was always a nurse on the ward, so there would always be someone around to help and advise. She then went on to explain that I would probably fall quite ill the following week. I wouldn't be back for my next cycle for another two weeks, and in that time patients normally catch an infection and have treatment for it in their local hospital before they return for the next lot of chemo. I sat trying to take everything in, but I was still so tired from all the treatment. I tried hard to concentrate as the nurse explained that the chemo causes the blood cell count to fall and as a result of this your immune system to drop. I would be most vulnerable to infections and illness in about ten days, and I should try to protect myself as much as possible, stay away from people with colds, not share drinks with anyone, and so on. When your blood cell count is at its lowest, and you are most vulnerable, they say you're neutropenic. The nurse told my mum that if I got ill in about a weeks time, it would probably be because I was neutropenic and had caught an infection from somewhere. She said that often, no matter how hard you try to look after yourself, it's impossible to avoid infections, and that she should take me straight to my local hospital and tell them I was neutropenic so they could get me into an isolation room as quickly as possible to avoid further illness. It all sounded a bit dramatic, and I lay back on the bed as the nurse tapped me on the leg and rubbed it, then carried on seeing to the other patients. It took an age for pharmacy to send up my medication, but as soon as I was handed the bulging plastic bag, we were out of there!

Although the nurse had explained all the possibilities of infection and illness that I should be aware of in a week's time when my blood cell count was low, I wasn't aware of how prone to infection I was already. I didn't realise I needed to start protecting myself immediately, and that I should have booked a cab home through the hospital rather than using public transport. Nobody told us that there was a transport department by one of the entrances to the hospital downstairs that was free to use and was really the best way for me to get home. Oblivious of this, as soon as the doctors had discharged me, mum and I grabbed our bags and headed for the tube station. During the journey home, I felt progressively worse, and after half an hour was absolutely dying to go to the loo from all those fluids being pumped into me all week! By the time we were on the over-ground train, the last leg of our journey, I just wanted my bed. I rested my head against the train window, and put my feet up on the seat beside me to support my stomach, which was churning over and over. I had just got comfortable and was starting to nod off when I felt a sharp jab on my shoulder. I looked up to see a very stern looking older woman staring down at me. "Put your feet down, I want to sit there," she barked at me. I looked at her and then scanned the rest of the carriage noticing all the empty seats, including the one opposite me next to my mum.

"Can't you sit somewhere else?" my mum asked defensively.

"No, I want to sit there", the woman abruptly replied.

I managed to reply feebly that I wasn't feeling too great, as I'd just been in hospital for a week having chemotherapy, thinking that after hearing this she might retreat and sit elsewhere. Instead she snapped back at me, "Oh well, we've all got problems". I put my feet down, and sat up. I was too exhausted to argue.

As soon as we got home, I went straight to bed. Every now and then mum came into my room to see if I wanted anything to eat or drink, but I was just too tired. I didn't do much for the next couple days, just rested. I texted my friends to say that I was home, and that one out of six cycles was over. "I'm nearly half way through" I joked. A couple texted back to say well done.

My best friend, Lucy, replied to my message saying, "That's great, I'll be round to see you tomorrow". I felt huge relief that I would finally have some sort of normality in my life. I thought about some films we could watch when she came round, I could have a moan at her about Pete, and find out what she had been up to. I didn't want to talk about the hospital, losing my hair, being unable to eat, or having to piss in a jug. I just wanted to be normal, and talk about normal things.

She was coming round at midday the next day, so that morning I dragged myself out of bed and into the bathroom. Mum ran me a bath with plenty of bubbles, as I watched the water rise I thought how good it felt not to be surrounded by jugs of other people's deposits, and as I placed the ends of my Hickman Line over the side of the bath tub, I lay back as much as I could without getting it wet and relaxed. I was too frightened to wash my hair, I was terrified it might start to fall out and I'd have huge patches when Lucy came round, so when I got out of the bath I got dressed, and gently brushed my hair back into a pony tail.

Mum put on some lunch for us for when Lucy arrived, and she tried hard not to fuss over me as I tried to hide my Hickman tubes, and packed away my medication, syringes and blood forms in a vain attempt to conceal any evidence of there being a sick person living here. I wanted no reminders while I was with my friend, just a bit of normality. But Lucy was so weird with me when she came round, she was anything but normal. I opened the door, and invited her in, so happy to see her. She handed me a box of chocolates and I thanked her for them not having the heart to tell her that having a piece of chocolate in my mouth was like chewing on a bar of metal. As I put them in the kitchen I smiled at mum, "Lucy brought you round a present", I laughed.

"Oh lovely!" she said, "and don't you be telling any of your friends you're going off chocolate, I could get used to all these tasty treats!"

As I walked back into the living room Lucy was sitting awkwardly at the edge of the sofa. "You ok?" I asked.

"Yeah, yeah", she laughed, "so how was it?"

"It was fine", I replied, "easy! Anyway, I got some films out last night, I've seen them all, but I love all of them which one do you want to watch?" I asked spreading out my collection of DVDs in front of her on the carpet. "I've got pop corn, and crisps, and mum's doing us some pasta", I went on.

"I'm not that hungry really, and I can't stay long" she cut in.

"Oh, ok", I said, a little surprised. I looked up at her as she kept staring at the top of my head.

"Has it started to fall out yet?" she asked looking around the side of my head. In that split second, I hated her. What sort of friend was she to come round here, say she couldn't stay long and start talking about the one thing I was dreading out of the whole experience. Of course she wouldn't have known how I felt about it because she had never asked, I hadn't spoken to her since the party. If she had returned any of the texts I had sent her from my bed in the ward, or if she had been to visit me in hospital she would have known I couldn't eat chocolate any more, and she would have known that now I was home I just wanted some normality. I didn't need her to be sitting here looking at my head waiting to see if my hair was about to drop out at any given second. We didn't speak much for the rest of the time she was there, she watched TV as mum and I ate lunch, then she texted her dad to come and pick her up. "Was lovely to see you!" and she grinned at me as she left.

"Yeah", I replied, not really sure what to make of what had just happened. I didn't speak to Lucy for a long time after that. I kept her updated with my trips to the Middlesex Hospital in London and our local hospital, Queen Mary's. I understood she couldn't make it all the way up to London to see me, but it upset me when I told her I was in the local hospital and she didn't even reply, let alone come up to see me. She was supposed to be my friend, I couldn't believe how badly she was letting me down, just when I needed her most. Gradually, I stopped telling her where I was and what was happening, I started to realise that she didn't care, and wasn't interested. That was a particularly painful thorn, and one that I just didn't see coming. Just a few months previously she had written a poem about friendship for an English class we had, she typed it up and printed out a copy for me. Above the poem she pasted a couple of photos of the two of us taken when we were at Rainbows together many years ago, she then framed it and gave it to me as a birthday gift. Now, it was like I just didn't exist, that was a bitter pill to swallow.

As promised, within a couple of days I had a visit from a Macmillan nurse, her name was Janet. I was asleep on the sofa as she knocked on the door, and as she came into the living room I reckon she could tell immediately by the look on my face that I wasn't too impressed at being woken up to be prodded about! When I think back at the visits those lovely Macmillan ladies paid me I'm absolutely mortified at the way I behaved. I was always exhausted from the treatment when they arrived two days after I came out of hospital, so I was always really cranky! I don't think any of them ever saw me in a good mood, not that I was rude or snapped at them, more that I just didn't speak to them! My poor mum would be chatting away as she made them tea while I sat staring at the floor, and when I think back I realise how they must have absolutely dreaded coming round, having to sit with me as I scowled my way through their visits. But they were always so lovely to me, and made sure I was feeling safe and looked after. They were also a great support to my mum, and reassured her every time they came round that if she had a question, or she was worried, or just generally needed a chat, that they were always at the end of the phone, day or night.

They are an amazing group of ladies, they were always there throughout the whole of my treatment, and never made me feel I was overreacting or being silly when we called them in the middle of the night. When they came to the house they would talk about their own families and lives, joke about how their lazy husbands were getting on their nerves, one of them shared the news that her son was getting married and she was expecting her first grandchild, and she brought photos on her next visit to show us the memories of her son's big day. It was the normality I craved for from my friends, conversations about something other than cancer, disease, illness; the subjects that haunted every corner of my house.

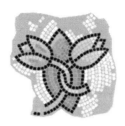

As I had been warned, I caught an infection the following week. I could feel myself burning up, and told mum I might need to go into hospital for some treatment. I was also really tired all the time, much more than when I was in hospital, I just couldn't keep my eyes open at all, and no matter how much I slept I was constantly tired when I woke up after a long nap. So mum took my temperature, and when it showed a high reading, bundled me into the car and took me to the local hospital. When we arrived we told the hospital that we thought I was neutropenic and had an infection. I was taken straight to an isolation room on a ward, I had no idea which one, all the corridors looked the same as I was being wheeled through them by the porter pushing my wheelchair. The nurses took some blood samples, but said from the look of me I probably needed a blood transfusion too. They said the telltale signs are feeling constantly sleepy, and having a really pale face, which I did. As I had a high temperature, they said it was almost certain I had an infection, so I was hooked up to some antibiotics, even though they couldn't be exactly sure what type of infection I had, nor where it was in my body. They explained that it is best just to start treating the infection as soon as possible, to prevent it from getting any worse, and as soon as my blood test results came in, confirming I had a low haemoglobin count, I was rigged up to a blood bag for a transfusion. My brother visited a little later that day and completely freaked out when he saw all the bags of blood I had lined up for me, a couple were empty, and a few were being prepared in case I needed more. "I can't feel it", I assured him when I saw the horrified look on his face, "it just goes through my Hickman, and I don't feel anything".

"Ok", he replied sounding unconvinced. After a few days I was feeling much better. The transfusions had made me feel a little ill after the first couple of bags of blood, but after taking two anti-sickness tablets before a third bag was fed through, I was absolutely fine. This is a breeze! I thought to myself, if all the infections are like this, I'll get through the next six months with no trouble at all! Oh, how wrong I was!

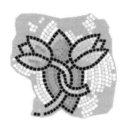

One morning during my second cycle, I was sitting on my hospital bed trying to get on with my school notes. I was having such difficulty concentrating; I wanted nothing more than to be in my classroom—strange as that sounds! The thought of studying along with the rest of my friends, as I did before any of this started, felt like a real treat. Instead, I was trying to teach myself from a distance, a load of information that my brain just pushed straight back out again. It was at times such as these, when I was trying to do my schoolwork, that I really missed my friends. But as time progressed they became increasingly distant. I texted them all the time, but they never replied. It was as if they had gone back to school after the summer break, and I was no longer part of the group. 'Out of sight, out of mind' they say, and that's exactly how I felt, so I gradually stopped communicating with them. It was heartbreaking every time I checked my phone and saw a blank screen, indicating that no one had returned my calls or messages. I was going through enough, I didn't need a dose of rejection on top.

Around midday the post arrived and I got a delivery! I certainly wasn't expecting anything so I thought it might have been a gift sent from one of the girls at school, or perhaps someone in the family. My eyes lit up as I looked at my mum, and I started tearing the parcel open. Inside was a plastic bag, and as I pulled it out and looked at it, my excitement turned to pure dread. I felt as though I had been punched in the stomach as the realisation of what had actually been sent to me set in. It was my token free wig, sent from the NHS. Here it was, staring me in the face, the one thing out of this entire experience that was haunting me the most; the fact that my hair was going to fall out. I held it up to examine it: the hair was short and curly, it was a sort of off-grey mousey brown colour, it was absolutely horrific. My eyes welled up as I stared down at the dead rat they expected me to put on my head, and wear in public. I put it back in the bag, placed the bag in the box, and silently gave it to a nurse to send back.

The hair was very obviously more appropriate for someone much older than I was. Apparently all the hair that was sent out was exactly the same. How ridiculous! As if the whole experience isn't bad enough, losing your hair and identity at such a sensitive age isn't undignified enough; being handed a substitute in this fashion just added salt to the wound. Seeing my pain, my mum suggested that we go shopping for some hair when I got out of hospital, and I agreed on the condition that I wasn't confronted with a specimen like that again! So I continued the cycle of treatment; the five days felt like five years, but I was finally allowed to go home.

A few days later, I built up the strength to go 'hair-shopping'. I was very aware that I was running out of time, my hair would fall out soon and I had no back up or scarves to wear when it did happen. So mum said she would take me to Oxford Street. She thought it would be a nice idea to take a look at what was on offer, and then treat me to some lunch. Grandad came along too, the sun was shining as we all strolled down the street to the station. Mum suggested we try one of the main department stores first; she had heard that one in particular had a special area that catered for people who had lost their hair and grandad told me not to worry about the price, that if I saw hair that I wanted I could have it. He knew how important it was to me that it looked as real and as natural as possible. Although I didn't live far from London, I hadn't ever been shopping in the West End before, and certainly hadn't been to the busy and bustling Oxford Street. Getting off the tube at Tottenham Court Road, we walked the whole street until we arrived at the department store mum had suggested. As we went in, I was actually filled with a little bit of excitement. I was sure I was going to find the perfect hair here, and I started to feel a little bit more relaxed about losing my own. Besides, nothing could be worse than the offering I had been handed the week before.

We were directed to the department we needed, and as we entered through the glass doors saw that it was tiny with a small old lady standing behind the counter. Her hair matched those on all the models behind her. I couldn't believe it, not again, and I felt that same kick to my stomach. Seeing my face drop, grandad asked politely, "Is that the extent of your variety? I think she's looking for something a bit longer, something that suits her age a bit more", his voice had a hopeful tone to it.

The old lady peered over her glasses at him, glanced at my mum, then at me, and then again at grandad before she replied sharply, "If you want a wig, that's all you're going to get". That was it, I was going home! I told mum and grandad to forget it, this was an impossible task. There was no way I was having granny-hair, I'd rather go out with no hair at all. On the way home I bought a few scarves to hide the fact that my own hair was starting to fall out at the top of my forehead. I could never get them to sit right though, and they'd often start to slip off because they were too small, but I managed with them for a while.

It wasn't until I was back in hospital for my next batch of chemo, that another patient's mum told us about a shop called Trendco. Every time I had been in for treatment, Lara was too, so our mums became quite friendly. Lara didn't wear any hair, she always opted for scarves instead, but someone else had told her about the little shop called Trendco in Kensington. Mum was telling her about our disastrous mission to find nice, realistic long hair for me, and Lara's mum asked if we had heard of the little shop. We said we hadn't, so she gave us the address, and showed us the samples of hair given to her by the patient who had recommended the shop. She said that she had never been, however, she had heard truly great things about it. I was very cautious; I didn't need to feel humiliated again. I thought it would be better to just leave it, besides, Lara always looked stunning with just her simple scarves on, so I would just do the same. But mum knew how much I was dreading being bald, so she encouraged me to take one last chance and go with her to Kensington. I agreed, reluctantly.

Once again, after my week's treatment was completed, mum, grandad and I continued my search for nice hair, and so we went to Kensington. It took what felt like forever to find the shop, but when we came across it, it was small, discreet and very welcoming. As we entered, an enthusiastic assistant immediately greeted us, and he offered us drinks and refreshments. After the long journey and anticipation of getting there, I would have very much appreciated a large vodka along with the orange juice I accepted; to my disappointment, this was not on offer. I explained why we had come to the shop, and as I was telling him about my treatment I glanced over his shoulder and saw a jaw-dropping array of models and hair. Different styles, shades and lengths; all made from either acrylic or human hair. I couldn't believe it; I was so unimaginably relieved that my eyes filled with tears. The assistant mistook my tears for those of sadness. He rushed to comfort me, telling me that this would only be a temporary replacement for my real hair, that my own would grow back soon. But they were not tears of sadness, they were tears of pure relief; I knew that we had finally come to the right place. He immediately ushered me towards the back of the shop, which had been set up just like a hair salon. There were a few individual cubicles lined up next to one another, each with its own mirror and chair—just like at the hairdressers! He sat me down in front of the mirror and tied the hair I had remaining up into a net on the top of my head. He saw that my hair was auburn and asked if I wanted my 'new hair' to be as similar to my own as possible. I looked at my mum as I said, "Yes"; I couldn't believe what I was hearing after all this time! This place was incredible. At my lowest point, and at the stage I was dreading the most, for the hour or so I was in the shop, I felt so dignified, so comfortable. What a contrast to how I felt looking down at the hair from the NHS on the ward that day, and those on offer in the department store a few weeks before. The assistant disappeared into the main part of the shop, and returned after a couple of minutes holding a long, auburn silky piece of hair. I didn't need to see any others, I knew that this was the one; it was perfect. He stood behind me as he arranged it on my head. It was synthetic, but still had a light fringe and parting, so it looked very realistic. I just couldn't believe it; it looked exactly like my own hair. The assistant then brushed it, and trimmed it around the front so that the hair framed my face—just as though I was in an actual hairdressers! He fluffed it and feathered it, all the time repeating the word 'fabulous' over and over.

"You look fabulous, darling, fabulous, it just works, you know. It works", he said, until by the end of our session I actually felt fabulous—for the first time in a long time. Looking at myself in the tiny cubicle with fading eyebrows and almost no eyelashes he still managed to make me feel beautiful. My grandad paid, and as I stepped out of the shop door, the sun was shining on my face and I felt the weight of the world lift from my shoulders.

When I talk about my hair falling out, and having to buy new hair, I tend not to use the word 'wig'. I don't use it because I don't like it. I think it sounds old fashioned, it automatically makes me think of short, grey curly hair, similar to those we saw at the department store on Oxford Street. I hate saying it and all words associated with it, so instead I gave my hair a name—Jemima. And from that day on Jemima and I went everywhere together! She gave me confidence to go out, to dress up, to be normal, to be—fabulous!

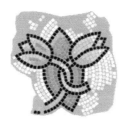

It was pitch black. I woke up dying to use the loo, so I jumped out of bed and ran next door to the bathroom. I felt my way into the room, reluctant to turn the light on so as not to wake the rest of the house, and I could feel my face starting to burn up. As I sat on the loo, all the familiar symptoms of an infection hit me, consumed me like a wave drowning me. As my eyes started to adjust to the darkness around me, I could feel my pulse thumping against my head, and my palms starting to sweat. I thought about waking mum up, dreading another midnight dash to A&E, when I was distracted by the sound of a really low-flying airplane. I looked up and out of the window behind me. I froze. The noise got louder as I watched a World War Two German jet fighter plane descending towards me. I ducked, it was flying so low I was convinced it was going to hit the house. I was so frightened. Cowering, I kept an eye on it as at it slowly steered upwards and missed the house. There was an almighty crash as it clipped the chimney on the roof, but the plane looked unscathed as I watched bricks falling past the window, tumbling down towards the ground. I screamed for mum. As I ran out of the bathroom and into her room I could hear the drone of the planes as the bombs dropped from the skies, narrowly missing our house each time. "Mum, mum! What are we going to do?" I screamed at her. But she was so calm, if not a little annoyed.

"What are you talking about?" she replied, her voice stern.

"What?!" I was panicking, "the bombs! They're going to hit us! We don't have anywhere to go, we need to get away from them, we don't have a shelter! What's going on?" But mum turned over in her bed and lay with her back to me.

"Go back to sleep, stop being so ridiculous!" she replied already half asleep. I was so confused. I looked up at the window; the street was lit up by flames, the noise was deafening, why was she telling me to go back to bed? Bewildered, I did what she said. I lay there, so still, surrounded by the sounds of bombs destroying the little town I grew up in, accompanied by the sounds of my neighbours screaming as they ran out of their houses not knowing what to do, where to go, who to ask for help. I was terrified as I lay back and closed my eyes. The tears streamed down my face, when as suddenly as it had started, the noise stopped. There were no more low-flying planes soaring past my window, and my bedroom no longer lit up each time a bomb fell outside in the street. I sat up and peered out of the window from behind my curtain. The street was so still, the ground was undisturbed and the stars were shining so brightly in the sky, with not a single plane in sight ruining my view of the heavens. I ran to the bathroom again, this time to be sick.

Mum sleepily came into the bathroom behind me, and started to rub my back. "What was all that about?" she asked. I sat on the floor looking at her, but couldn't answer her. I had seen the planes and the bombs so clearly, I had ducked when I thought the planes were about to hit the house, I shielded my eyes each time the street lit up from the blaze of each bomb. Yet now, not five minutes later everything was so still, so peaceful.

I was getting sick for a while, so mum said we'd run up to the hospital first thing in the morning. Things calmed down for the rest of the night, I was still being sick regularly, but at least the Germans were no longer attacking. I was so confused, and so very frightened. What was happening to my mind? It definitely hadn't been a dream—after all, I had woken mum up so I had to have been awake. Perhaps I was sleepwalking, but even to this day I can see so clearly the destruction and the war zone the street had turned into. In my mind, it's still as if it all happened yesterday. This bloody chemo is actually driving you mad I thought to myself as I watched my mum gather some things together ready to take me to the local hospital, Queen Mary's.

I kept my pyjamas on. I couldn't be bothered to get dressed. As I cleaned my bucket ready for the road again, mum called grandad to let him and nan know that we were on our way to the hospital. We arrived at A&E, and I started to feel dizzy. I was brought straight up to a ward and put on a drip. The doctors explained that because I had been getting sick all night, I needed to be given fluids straight away, to re-hydrate. Then I slept. I slept for hours, with mum by my bedside, as usual. When I woke they told me I had septicaemia, "Isn't that really bad?" I asked, trying to sit up.

"It can be", the doctor replied, "but we've caught it in time, you just need plenty of rest".

The doctor then gave me a quick examination, he checked my mouth, my ears, and tested my reflexes. He then asked how long I had been feeling unwell for. I explained that the night before I had been feeling a bit dizzy and been sick. I told him about the German planes I had seen so vividly, and the bombs that lit up the street as they exploded. He smiled and sat down on the bed beside me. "They were hallucinations you were experiencing", he began to explain.

"But it was all so vivid", I told him, "I could hear the bombs dropping, the neighbours screaming". He nodded and went on to say that sometimes a clip on TV, or something someone said in passing can trigger off such visions. I tried to think back over all the conversations I had had the day before. I remembered sitting in my grandad's front room the previous evening, we had just got in from church and we all sat down in front of the TV to hear the news. There was a breaking story, America had attacked Iraq in the still of the night. We watched the TV footage of the Iraqi countryside being lit up as the bombs fell from the skies.

"It's World War Three", grandad said.

'You'll often have nightmares," the doctor's voice took me away from grandad's living room, "and although you may wake up in the middle of a nightmare," he warned, "it can continue as a hallucination so you need to try and snap yourself out of it". How am I supposed to do that? I thought to myself, I couldn't understand what he was saying.

"Surely when it seems so real, it'll be impossible to snap myself out of it" I replied, "I got so angry with mum when she wouldn't get up and just lay in bed while our entire road was being destroyed around us. I was so frightened, and she did nothing". The doctor turned to speak to my mum, she was standing at the bottom of my bed with a horrified look on her face. He explained to her that, most of the time, it's best for the person having the hallucination if people around them go along with it and agree with what they think they can see. Having such a violent and vivid vision is terrifying, they need to be comforted and assured that they are safe without the added fear that they're going mad. They need to be told that the things they can see won't harm them and will soon pass, or leave them alone. Mum started to get upset, she thought she had done the wrong thing and made me feel worse. I told her to stop being silly, and gave her a cuddle as the doctor left the room to continue his ward round. Then I had a thought. How funny that medication, which is supposed to make you better, can make you feel worse than when you started the treatment! It brings on such dangerous and violent illnesses, with terrifying side effects. How ironic it seems, that rather than the cancer, it could in fact be the chemo, intended to save you, that kills you.

"Do not watch the petals fall from the Rose with sadness, know that, like life, things sometimes must fade, before they can bloom again"

Anon

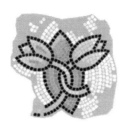

I was midway through my treatment. As the medication took hold, I noticed that my hair wasn't the only thing being affected by the toxic medication. I guess because my main concern was losing my hair, and it was really all I spoke or asked about, the hospital team had bypassed everything else that comes along with it. I hadn't been warned about the other ways chemo would affect my appearance and my body, and I was frightened when I began to notice changes. I worried that perhaps I was having an extreme reaction, and that these changes would never rectify themselves. I remember waking one morning to find my entire face, neck, back and even my scalp covered in tiny spots. I was 16 so admittedly I was used to one or two! I had become an expert at covering up the odd one when they broke out because of stress, or because it was 'lady time'. But this was absolutely horrific. I screamed for my mum as I stood in the bathroom horrified at my reflection. She just looked at me; I looked like something from a horror film, and she told me to get in the car and we went straight to A&E at Queen Mary's Hospital, I was becoming a bit of a regular there now! At the hospital, they took me straight to an isolation room while I waited for a doctor. The ward nurse popped in while I sat on the bed running my fingers through my hair and feeling a few strands come out in my hand each time. The nurse was male, and the absolute double of Elvis. He came equipped with the quiff and even had the collar on his uniform turned up as he swaggered into the room. I knew immediately that he was going to irritate me. He came over to me, looked at my face, and said, "It's a bad case of acne, you're a teenager, and you've got spots. What a surprise!" I was right, he was getting on my nerves already.

"I've never had spots this bad" I protested, "maybe the odd one or two, but this is all over my scalp as well!"

"Well, get used to it", he said "this is gonna last for at least the next few years", and with that, he swaggered back out.

"He's going to get a thick lip if he comes back in here" was my mum's response. I had to laugh. My mum is the most placid lady you'll ever meet, she's tiny and very feminine, so hearing her 'fighting talk' had me on the floor. It was probably the first time I had laughed in quite a while, and as we were giggling, a doctor walked in. He looked puzzled, and said he had never experienced a reaction to chemo like this before. I started to panic, but he assured me that everyone reacts differently to treatment. He prescribed some cream, and instructed me to use it on my face, neck and back.

"But what about my head?" I asked. My hair was starting to fall out, which was bad enough, but I didn't want my scalp to be covered in these awful blemishes. "Well, just see how you get on with the cream, and we'll go from there", he replied. I took the cream, thanked him, got down from the bed and left.

I was feeling so exhausted from the treatment, as soon as I got in I applied the cream as he had said, and went straight to sleep. I must have been really tired, as I didn't wake until the next morning. The sunlight streaming through the curtains woke me. I lay in my bed for some time that morning, thinking about the state of my face and imagining the scarring that would be left when it eventually cleared up. I wondered what other conditions and ailments the chemo would bring, and how long I would have to wait for my hair to fall out completely. I asked myself, for the umpteenth time what had I done to deserve such a bad hand? What could I have done to prevent it? Fed up with feeling sorry for myself, I decided to get up and have a look in the mirror to see what the damage to my face was this morning. I couldn't believe what was looking back at me. My skin was completely clear, not a single blemish was visible. I turned to look at my back, and that too had cleared up. I ran my fingers through my hair and could feel my scalp was completely smooth. I was so relieved I sat on the bathroom floor, and cried.

With time, I also noticed my nails were gradually weakening. They would bend and break much more than usual. I thought perhaps I needed to up my calcium intake, but no matter how much milk I drank, or supplements I took, nothing seemed to help. Eventually, they fell off. The same sinking feeling I had when I saw my skin had broken out, hit me again. I was so horrified at the state of my ugly hands that I immediately made an appointment at my local nail bar, and I went with a friend to have false ones put on. But as the nail technician was primping and buffing what little was left of my own nails, the pain became unbearable. I winced through the agony as she finished putting on the last nail, and before they even had a chance to properly set I paid and ran out of the shop. Although they were much prettier to look at than what was hidden underneath, the false nails were mostly attached to raw skin. I couldn't bear to keep them on for longer than a day, and it was absolute agony trying to remove them from the thin layer of damaged skin beneath them where my own nail should have been. But what upset me most wasn't the pain, or even the fact that my nails had gone, instead I was deeply saddened at the way I was trying, and failing, to make myself look and feel better in the face of what I was going through. Despite how the treatment was affecting my body, I was trying so desperately to cover it up. I just wanted to be a pretty, attractive, normal 16 year old, with nice nails, hair and complexion. I was fed up trying to hide the parts of me that might give away the type of treatment I was having, but I was getting tired of fighting a losing battle.

The next change I noticed was to my skin. My arms and tummy started to turn, what I can only describe as, scaly, a bit like a reptile's. It looked yellow, and flaky, a bit like eczema I guess. Again, I tried to cover it up, using creams, lotions and moisturisers, but nothing worked. Nothing I could think of removed or hid the scale-like patterns on my skin, so instead I covered myself up all the time, I made sure I kept all of my arms and legs covered despite it being the middle of an absolutely gorgeous summer.

Along with these side affects, my mouth also started to suffer. I developed ulcers along my gums and along the roof of my mouth. The hospital provided me with several mouthwashes and drinks to try to prevent, or at least heal them. As an open wound, they were a risk of infection, so I used the mouthwash religiously, even though it tasted horrendous, and really discoloured my teeth! But my cuts and ulcers were made a hundred times worse by the braces

I had had fitted a few months before I was diagnosed. My consultant advised that I have them removed prematurely, as it may make life a bit more bearable, and give my mouth a chance to heal in-between chemo doses. I started to feel increasingly angry at the treatment rather than the actual disease. It was stripping away every part of me, and my identity. I tried so hard to combat the side effects, and fight what the medication was doing to my body, but it was an impossible battle. I realised again that, yes, it was saving my life, but hand-in-hand with this it was making me so ill. And it was even harder for me to accept that it would all eventually be worth it the day my hair fell out.

As the weeks throughout my treatment passed, I could feel strands of hair falling out. It felt like a kick to the stomach the first time I ran my fingers through my hair and was left with a bundle of it in my hand. I tried to convince myself that it was no more than what might normally come out when you ruffle you hair, but I knew deep down it was really happening now. I prayed that this would be it, just a few strands here and there, that way perhaps I'd at least be able to cover up any small gaps with the rest of my hair. I prayed every day that it wouldn't fall out, and for a while to my relief, it was just a few strands here and there. I remember getting ready to go to church one Sunday, I was absolutely terrified to wash my hair before we went, I knew it wouldn't be long now, and I had an awful feeling that as soon as I lay back in the bath it would all fall out at once. I wasn't ready, but in the same breath, I knew I would never be ready for this. There would never be a right time to lose my hair, to be bald, and I hated it, I felt angry, I felt robbed of a normal life. I massaged the shampoo and conditioner into my hair so gently, and took my time washing it out. I panicked when I felt strands coming out in my hands, and as I lay in the bath, stared at them floating on the water's surface. It took a couple of hours in all to wash, comb and blow dry my hair, for what turned out to be the last time. I wanted so badly to show every one that I was still beautiful. I wanted people to remember me as, Natasha, and not 'you know, that girl with cancer'. So I carefully finished styling my hair, and put on a dress. It was purple with pink and gold lining, knee length and gorgeous. I left the house with my head held high. Mum and I got into my little metro, and she drove the five minute journey to church. After the service I spoke to some friends, everyone said how well I looked, but inside I was crumbling. The more I touched my head throughout the service, the more hair came out in my hands, but I managed to keep myself together until I got home. My eyes filled with tears as I showed my mum how easily my hair was now falling out, but what could she say to me? She just held me as tears fell down my cheeks. We snuggled on the sofa that evening, as the reality of what this treatment was doing to me really started to hit home.

That night I felt really ill. I lay in bed and could feel my temperature rising. My throat hurt and I was getting more and more irritable. Suddenly I started to really shiver. I had gone from burning up to feeling absolutely freezing, but was still sweating at the same time. I lay shuddering under my covers as I called for my mum. As she came into my room I asked her to put the heating on. I couldn't understand how the temperature in the house could have dropped so suddenly and so quickly, my teeth were chattering as I spoke to her. Mum tucked me into bed tightly and went to make me a cup of tea to warm me up. She knew something must have been wrong, as she hadn't noticed a change in the temperature, and yet I was obviously so cold. When she came back with the tea, she had a thermometer with her as well. The hospital told us that anything between 36°C and 37°C was normal, and to get in touch with my local hospital if it was any different. Expecting it to be lower than 36°C because I was shivering so much, we were both shocked when the tiny screen on the side of the thermometer read 39.9°C! Mum was so confused, how could I be so cold, yet have a reading that was so high? So she phoned my Macmillan nurse. What a life-line those nurses were. 'Call anytime you need us', they told us when we were first introduced at the beginning of my treatment, and that night at three in the morning, they were at the end of the phone immediately, just as they had promised. They explained that the high temperature reading indicated that I had a bad infection, but I was shivering so violently because it is the body's way of trying to cool itself down. They told mum to get me to the hospital immediately, not to wait for an ambulance, but to take me there herself as it would be quicker. They also told her to take the bedclothes off me, as I needed to shiver to cool myself down. My poor mum; she hung up the phone, grabbed a bag and threw some pyjamas, a toothbrush and some underwear into it. She then came into my room and explained that we had to get to the hospital quickly, helping me out of bed and down the stairs to the car as she spoke. I was trying to take the duvet with me, but mum was gently pulling it away following the advice the nurse had given her. So we fought with the bed covers all the way down the stairs to the car, until we compromised and she gave me a small blanket as I sat in the front seat shaking with the cold.

We arrived at Queen Mary's A&E department, with me drifting in and out of sleep. Because I was neutropenic the hospital staff were quick to rush me to a ward where they gave me a room to myself. My immune system was now so low, and I was very vulnerable to infections, I couldn't risk being on a ward with other patients, and so again I needed to be in isolation. Throughout the night and during the following day, many blood tests and scans were carried out on me. Quite often, when a patient develops an infection as a result of being on chemo, doctors are unable to identify the exact cause of the infection, however, a large dose of antibiotics is usually enough to calm the symptoms down and help the infection pass. On this occasion though the doctors were unable to identify the problem, and the antibiotics they had administered were having absolutely no effect. My heart was racing, and the hospital staff were becoming increasingly concerned throughout the day, as more medication proved unsuccessful. But they kept trying, doing more and more blood tests and giving me more and more antibiotics in an attempt to calm the infection's symptoms down. Eventually they discovered I had meningitis. They diagnosed it just in time before it was able to cause any serious, permanent damage. I knew from the reaction of the doctors things were bad, their sense of urgency was frightening, no matter how hard they tried to cover it up. I knew also that if mum had left it until the morning to call the nurse and tucked me in tightly for the night, things would be very different now. Once again, she had saved my life.

Finally, on the correct medication, I was comfortable enough to sleep for the rest of the day. Family came and went, they brought tea and fruit with them for mum, and tried to persuade her to go home with them to get some rest now that I was getting a bit better. But she stayed by my side, staring at the four walls and refusing to leave until I woke the following morning.

I woke feeling so much better, I felt refreshed and relieved to be neither sweating nor shivering. Mum asked me if I fancied something small to eat; my mouth was in agony from all the tiny little cuts that had developed around my gums, but I was so hungry, I asked for anything she could find that was soft. So she popped downstairs for some fresh air, a couple of bananas for us and some more magazines. While I waited, my head still cushioned by a few pillows, I switched the TV at the bottom of my bed on and relaxed. Being on chemotherapy caused my concentration span to become quite short, and I was finding it hard to focus on one programme for more than 15 minutes, so I put the music channels on instead. Watching the sexy young pop stars do their thing on the screen, I found myself singing along to the music videos. To my amazement, I realised the chemo had also affected my voice. I could hear myself croaking along to the songs, and found I wasn't able to reach notes as high as I normally could. Just something else I would have to get used to I thought to myself.

Soon mum returned with some goodies, and although I was still a bit weak, I pulled myself up in the bed so that I could sit up straight and talk to her. It was a struggle though, my back and bum were really aching from lying down so much! As I sat up and reached for a banana in the bag mum had put at the end of my bed, her face fell. She was staring at me, and her eyes started to fill with tears. "Honey", she said, "your hair". I put my hand to my head and could feel my bare scalp. I turned in the bed to see that my hair had remained on the pillow as I sat up. It was that quick. I was speechless. I was still holding my head and staring at the pillow as a cleaner walked into the room, whistling and sweeping the floor as he entered.

"Don't worry love", he sang to me, "it'll grow back!" I just sat and stared at him, with my mouth open, and my hand resting on the bare skin where my long auburn hair should have been. He left as quickly as he came in, leaving mum and I just looking at each other. She came over to me and sat next to me on the bed. She held me, and rocked me as I cried on her shoulder. She held me like I was her little girl again, at what was probably the lowest moment of my treatment. What could she say to me now? What could she do? Kiss me on the forehead and make it all better again? I pulled away from her and stood up next to the bed. I walked over to the sink in the corner of the room, which had a mirror fixed to the wall above it. So there I was, face to face with my nightmare—the one thing that had haunted me since the day I had been diagnosed. Other than a few whispy strands left at the back of my head, and behind the tops of my ears, I was bald.

Looking back, perhaps it had been a good thing that it all fell out at once. At least this way, I hadn't gone through the torment that some experienced of it thinning and fading away, neither did I have to make the tough decision of shaving it off if a large patch had appeared. It was still hard though—my toughest battle. The most painful thorn on my rose had well and truly stung me.

I spent the remainder of the week in Queen Mary's. My braces were causing so much pain rubbing against the sores in my mouth that mum arranged for my Orthodontist to come to the hospital to remove them in my little room. She was a really stern woman, very direct and not particularly delicate when you were sitting in her chair! But when she arrived that day I saw a completely different side to her. She explained that she was unable to bring the appropriate equipment with her to remove the braces, so she would have to make do with trying to prise them off with the utensils she could bring. Great! I thought, as if all this wasn't painful enough! But she was lovely, as she tried to make the procedure as painless as possible, and she gave me a little hug as she left. When she had gone, I sat and reflected on my journey so far: I was bald, scaly, had wonky, discoloured teeth and no nails! Not great! But I had determination enough to get through all of it, and more importantly, I had the unquestioning support of my lovely family.

I was discharged that Friday night, and so I had the weekend at home before I had to return to the Middlesex Hospital for my next lot of treatment the following Monday morning. But it wasn't until I was leaving my hospital room and had to walk through the children's ward towards the exit, that I saw all the other patients. I had always been rushed in and out of the ward in Queen Mary's, so I hadn't paid much attention to the other patients I shared the wards with, but for some reason on this occasion, I looked into the main bays as we walked towards the exit. I was absolutely heartbroken. I saw toddlers, and new-born babies attached to drips and blood bags via their tiny Hickman Lines. Some were cuddling teddy bears that had their own little Hickman lines sellotaped to their furry tummies, others were just screaming with pain unable to communicate where it was coming from, or how ill they felt. Instead, they had to rely on their frantic parents' intuition and instincts. Born fighting, how unfair it seemed that they had to start life this way.

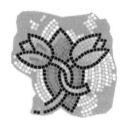

When I think of my mother, my most poignant memories are of a time that must have been very uncertain for her. My dad had just left the two of us, along with my precious newborn baby brother. He left us for another woman, for another family. It must have left my mum shattered, insecure, vulnerable and desperate. But to me, she has never been more beautiful. When I think of her picking herself and two tiny children up; fighting through the heartbreak; collecting the pieces of our little broken family, and carefully putting us back together, I see her strength and the unconditional love only a mother can give.

As soon as I was diagnosed, mum asked me if I wanted to get in touch with my dad, I guess to let him know what was happening. At the time I was taken aback a little, it came completely out of the blue, but I know now she was thinking ahead, she worried in case I might need some form of transplant, fearing that he would be the only match for me. She was also concerned that he or his family might have some medical history that the doctors would need to know about, something that might give them some indication as to why this had happened to me. I can't imagine the courage it must have taken for her to ask me this, knowing there was a huge chance I might have said 'yes, I want to find him, I need all the support I can get'. But I know without a doubt, that if I had have asked her to put some form of search in motion, she'd have done it. Without blinking an eye she would have tracked him down for me, because I had asked her to. As it turned out, I looked at her completely confused. "Why would I want that mum?" I asked, "I have all the support I need right here. We haven't needed him up to now have we? We'll be fine! If I need help, a transplant, or blood, or anything else, I'd rather accept it from a complete stranger than take anything from him. I don't want to owe him anything, now, that's enough of that".

The truth of it is I didn't need anyone else. Nan, grandad, mum and Dom, they were my pillars of strength, they got me through my darkest days. They also did some pretty crazy stuff for me too throughout the treatment. As the chemo really affected my taste buds, I started to ask for food I normally didn't really like and hadn't really eaten before, pizza being one of them, although I still love it! Mum would worry when I hadn't eaten all day while the chemo was being fed through my Hickman Line, it would get to the evening, and she'd ask me to eat something, just a little bit of anything. I couldn't touch anything from the hospital food trolley as was the case with most of the patients, so every night mum would run around the streets getting take-ways from different restaurants for me. In a week, I'd be presented with cuisine from around the globe, one night it would be pizza or pasta, then fish and chips, kebabs, curries. My mouth would water at the thought of her bringing in a doner kebab with all the trimmings and sauce, and I'd ask her to be as quick as she could. Usually,

I would see what someone else on the ward was eating and get a little envious, and other times, all the mums would get together and get fish and chips or pizza for everyone and we'd all sit talking together and sharing. That was the lovely thing about that ward, every one was in the same boat, we were all sailing up shit creek, but we were sailing it together. Unfortunately though, quite often by the time mum had come back with the food, I had gone off it and fancied something else instead, just as the dietician had warned us. It would happen that quickly, mum would walk into the ward with a chicken curry and the smell of it would make me physically sick, and she would often end up giving my food to other patients, or their visitors. That's how people become so weak and fragile on chemo, it's not a case of being fussy, as I often felt I was being, the smells and taste of foods become so different and often so awful in a split second, you simply cannot eat it.

In my local hospital though, things were a bit better as I wasn't having my chemotherapy there so didn't go off food so much, but it was still an issue. Because I was in having treatment for an infection, I was usually so weak, the food was terrible and being on a children's ward too, the portions were tiny! But once again, my crazy family came to the rescue. Queen Mary's was only ten minutes from nan and grandad's house, and every evening grandad would come to visit. He'd stay with me while mum and Dominic went off to have a coffee and a chat about how his day at school had gone, Grandad would always bring a plate of food that nan had just cooked with him. She'd warm the plate, dish up the food and put tin foil over the top to keep it warm, so it was still piping hot when he came rushing through the ward and into my room. I'd eat like a Queen, feasting on roasts, fish fingers, chips and beans, sausage, mash, peas, and gravy. How it didn't spill all over the car I'll never know, but I was always so grateful to see him arrive with a plate, I'd sit up in the bed and gobble it down in silence, mopping up the plate with my fingers when it was all gone. Then he'd take it back off me, run it under the tap in the sink beside my bed wrap it up with tissue and take it away with him. My lovely family, I would have been lost without them.

I missed the Teenage Cancer Trust Unit at the Middlesex when I was fighting infections in Queen Mary's in Sidcup. No matter how much I would moan about the smell, the food, and the smell *of* the food, it was a much nicer place to be. It was lively, there was always music playing, and we had a lovely activities co-ordinator, who was always encouraging us to make, paint or design things, just to take our minds off the treatment and our attention away from the constant bleeping of the machines around us. I didn't appreciate the work she did at the time, or how hard her job must have been, facing young sick people every day and trying to motivate them. The chemo always knocked me out, so I was never interested in making things, or decorating the area around my bed, and I was usually in a foul mood anyway so couldn't understand the point of it, or why any of the other patients would want to take part either. But now I see how important it was for some of the other patients to have something else to focus on, and it no doubt stopped them being a big grump like I was! One week, I was in the middle of a chemo cycle, and the activity co-ordinator organised a band to come into the ward. They were a percussion group, and performed all afternoon for the patients, and then gave us a chance to join in and have a go on their instruments. Before they arrived, the co-ordinator ran around each of the beds, trying to get us excited and ready for their visit, I love music so really tried hard to stay awake, but I just couldn't do it. I slept through the whole lot, I didn't even see the musicians arrive, let alone hear any music or have a go myself. Although, actually, that's not strictly true, I did contribute in my own way. As they finished one piece and were about to start another, silence filled the air keeping the ward in suspense, and with perfect timing I let out a huge snore! My poor mum nearly threw herself under the bed as all the eyes in the ward shot across the room to where we were, "Sorry", she mumbled, "you know how the chemo knocks her out!" Disgusted at my lack of appreciation of their art, they continued to entertain the rest of the patients until evening, what a shame I didn't get to see any of it!

But I had been warned that the chemo might make me very tired, and I appreciated the fact that it made me more sleepy than sick. Often, I'd drift off late morning and wake up in the middle of the afternoon, and only because I was dying to use the loo! I missed so many visits from family, I would wake up and mum would tell me who was here, and what they were saying. I felt bad for not being able to stay awake for just a couple of hours to talk to people who had made such an effort to come all the way up to London to see me. When I woke up I'd be surrounded by cards, or fruit and sweets and I'd know I'd slept through another visit. Sometimes I'd wake up and mum wouldn't be in her normal spot in the chair next to my bed reading a newspaper, and I'd panic. If I thought she was taking longer than a normal trip to the loo, or I couldn't hear her chatting to one of the other mums in the TV room, I'd ask the nurses where she had gone and why she wasn't coming back. Of course she was never far, most of the time, because I slept so much, when someone came to visit she would go to one of the cafés on the street outside for a quick coffee and a chat, but I hated it and I wanted her to come back straight away. I soon realised that I had come to rely very heavily on my mum, which must have put a lot of pressure on her. My independence was being snipped away by this drug, I couldn't bathe by myself in case I fell, I couldn't dress myself because my Hickman would get entangled without someone holding it away from my clothes, I always needed someone around, and that someone was always mum. Not only did cancer steal my life from me for those months, it stole hers too.

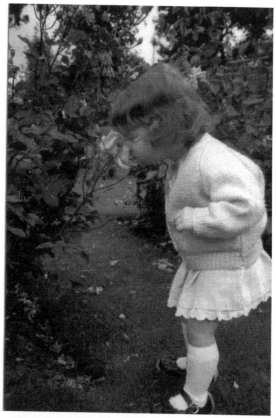

'Kissed By A Rose'—Aged Three in Ireland.

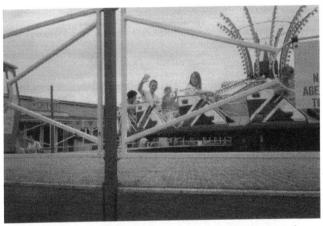

On one of many unbeatable holiday in Butlins with my lovely grandad.

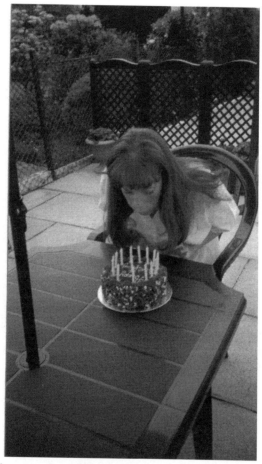

Celebrating my 15th Birthday, just months before the
biggest Thorn on my Rose stung.

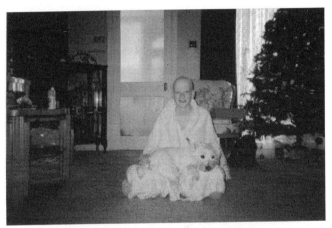

My biggest battle—losing my hair

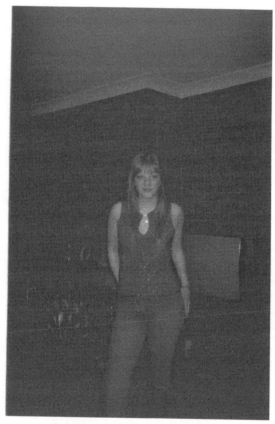

Jemima and I on a good day!

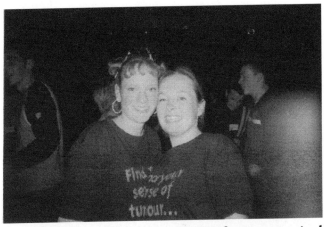

At a 'Find Your Sense of Tumour' Conference organised
by the Teenage Cancer Trust, with Rebecca.

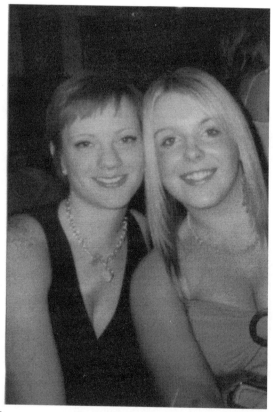

After my second round of chemo—with better hair, and better friends.

Louise, Me, Grace, Rebecca, Justine and Katharine, our roses have blossomed together.

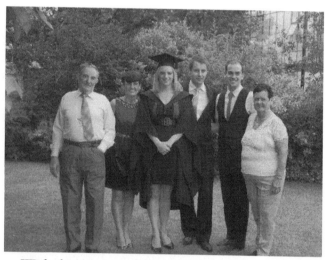

With the support of my mum, Dominic, nan and grandad, and with Andreas by my side, I finally got there!

"Silently one by one, in the infinite meadows of heaven Blossomed the lovely stars, the forget-me-nots, of angels"

Henry Wadsworth Longfellow

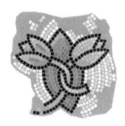

I don't think I'll ever really be able to adequately express the mixture of feelings and emotions that run through me when I think of the teenagers I have met who have lost their battle. The immense feeling of guilt I carried, that I survived and they didn't often consumed me. This was juxtaposed with a determination to fight the disease and spread a little bit of awareness that cancer in teenagers does exist, it was a confusing combination of emotions that has never really gone away. But I want to encourage young people to stand up for themselves when a GP tells them their symptoms and pains are in their head, or that they are simply looking for a bit of attention. Whether they think there might be something wrong with their leg, head, back, neck, balls, whatever; we can't afford to be embarrassed to talk about it anymore. If many of the teenagers that I met along this journey had been diagnosed sooner, perhaps they wouldn't be sitting amongst the stars now. I remember being in the waiting room, at my first follow-up appointment after all my chemo was all done and I was getting my first set of scan results whilst being in remission. It sounds crazy, but I kept thinking that it wouldn't be so bad if they came back showing another tumour, at least then I wouldn't feel like I had it so easy compared to the others. I hadn't lost a leg, I hadn't lost the use of any of my limbs, I hadn't lost my sight or any of my other senses, I hadn't lost my life. Why should I have got away with it so easily when so many others had suffered so much more?

When I think of Maggie, I see her smile. She always seemed so happy and I could never understand it. Our chemo cycles would often coincide so I pretty much saw her each time I was having my treatment. She was a tall, slim, brunette and absolutely stunning. When she was in for treatment everyone knew she was around, there was always a happy atmosphere, she was always so positive. I never got the feeling that she was feeling low, or having a bad day, although I'm sure she had many. Often, I'd sit on my bed across the other side of the ward from her just watching everyone. I'd usually be in a foul mood from the moment I stepped onto the ward until the second I left, and I'd sit and look at Maggie, who was always doing some sort of artwork or making jewellery. I'd think, 'what the hell has she got to smile about? Look where we are, what we're being forced to go through'. Of course it wasn't until she had gone that I realised how much I actually appreciated the way her smile brightened up the ward and I missed being woken up by her crazy laugh no matter what time it was. It was her 20th birthday during one of our cycles. "What a lovely way to spend the day, being stuck in here," I said to her sarcastically.

"It was bloody great! You know Oxford Street's only round the corner, I've been there all day!" She said, giving me a beautiful smile. She left me stunned as she went back to the treasures she had bought which were all laid out on her bed. Amongst them was a gorgeous pair of new knee-high boots that her parents had bought her earlier in the day. She then turned the ward into a catwalk, and proceeded to parade up and down in front of our beds making sure we were all watching her strut her stuff. Now, Maggie's tumour was in her leg, her knee specifically. She walked with quite a limp, so you can imagine what we all thought when she unveiled her boots from their box! But she didn't care. She threw them on, stood up, grabbed hold of her drip for support and she worked that catwalk while the rest of us clapped and cheered. After a while, we began to spend quite a lot of time together. Often our mums would go out and get some dinner for the two of us, and so we'd sit and eat together, and we'd compare symptoms and side effects. We'd reassure each other that we were doing fine, and share ideas and treatments that we found helped to combat the sickness we felt all the time. Sometimes I would come in for treatment wearing Jemima, and she always complimented me, so I told her about Trendco when she said she couldn't believe how realistic it looked. I hardly recognised her when I walked on to the ward at the Middlesex one day, she had been to Trendco herself, and she sat on her bed smiling at me with long, dark, shining, shimmering hair. She belonged on a catwalk. But after a while we started to see less and less of Maggie. I often asked about her, but patient confidentiality meant, the nurses' reply was always the same, 'Yeah, she's doing fine, she's getting on great!' Good, I'd think to myself, presuming our cycles had fallen out of sync, and we were just missing each other on the ward.

"Wouldn't it be lovely if the next time we see Maggie is when we're both in remission, attending clinic?" I said to mum as we left the hospital one day. Mum carried all our bags as we headed towards the hospital exit. Grandad had come to pick us up, and on this particular afternoon he had brought my nan with him. As we walked past the hospital chapel mum gave all the bags to grandad and asked him and nan to wait in the car for us.

"Come in here", she said, as she headed back down the corridor and in through the doors to the hospital chapel. How strange, I thought, we've been here all week and just as we're on the verge of escaping she decides that now's the time to say a little prayer! It was a tiny chapel, but the grandeur of the statues and altar more than made up for its size. We sat in a pew a few rows from the back, and mum took my hand. She looked at me with tears in her eyes, as she explained that the nurses had asked to her to break the news to me that Maggie had died a few days before.

"What are you talking about? I asked the nurses how she was, and they said she's fine! She's fine!" I shouted at her.

"No honey, she's gone, they asked me to tell you in our own time". The only emotion I remember feeling was anger. I was so angry with the world, life, God, everyone. Mum tried to comfort me, but I pushed her away. A beautiful young woman stolen away by this merciless disease. It didn't seem fair, she was always so positive, so keen to lift everyone else out of their sadness.

Soon after we left the hospital the guilt hit me like a brick in the face. I sat on my bed that evening, thinking about heaven's new angel. As I thought about what her family must be going through and how my mum would feel if I lost my battle, I decided I had to be a little more positive, after all, I wasn't in a box yet. Sort yourself out Tash, I thought to myself, this situation is shit for everyone, mum's hardly so much as smiled in weeks, Dominic's terrified every time you mention having a temperature. In that moment, I knew I needed to try to start living for the people who no longer had the chance.

I decided then, not to make any more good friends on the ward. I tried to be more positive, and always spoke to other patients giving them advice when I could, but I didn't allow myself to get close to anyone again, like I did with Maggie, the pain of losing another friend, I think would have been too much. Of course there were teenagers I saw each time I had my treatment—my cycle often coincided with a couple of the others. It was difficult not to become too friendly, because we shared such a unique experience, had the same illnesses, suffered the same torments. I'm sure for other people, making friends and having people they can truly confide in and spend time with at the hospital is what gets them through the treatment. But for me, and I can see that it's a very selfish emotion, I couldn't handle the guilt of surviving, when one of my friends didn't.

But I was always amazed at the courage other patients showed, like I say, my experience was mild compared to others, and I found it remarkable how some people were able to rise above what ever they were going though. Most people would use humour to overcome their fears, they would literally laugh in death's face as they joked around with hospital staff about what was happening to their bodies, stuff that was completely out of their control. One girl I saw quite often had a tumour in her leg. It was spreading from her thigh downwards, and nothing they could do was stopping it and containing it in one site, so the only option they had was to remove the whole leg. Throughout these months I thought about this a lot, amputation. My cancer was internal, in an organ that they were able to cut away at and reduce without too much complication, but what if it came back in my leg? My arm? What if I had to have something amputated, I'm not sure I could cope with that. I was in the bed beside hers the morning she went down for her operation. She was terrified, of course she was, but she was still laughing, and she wrote all the way down the infected leg, "IT'S THIS ONE! IT'S THIS ONE! IT'S THIS ONE!" and down the other leg, "NOT THIS ONE! LEAVE ME ALONE!" She waved goodbye to everyone saying she wouldn't be long, then they wheeled her out and down to surgery. I never saw her again.

There were a few side rooms at either end of the teenage ward. You had a room to yourself if you were particularly ill while having your treatment, or your immune system was very low and you were susceptible to picking up illnesses and infections from the other patients. Each time I was admitted for chemo, there was usually a guy, Adam, who was in one of side rooms recovering from infections. He was very ill, but still always such a 'geezer'! Although each time we saw him, his rose was fading in front of our eyes, his personality never withered. We got used to seeing him, and despite being very sick, he always made sure we were aware he was around! One afternoon I was sitting on my bed watching a DVD of 'Friends' on my laptop. Lunch had just been taken away, but the horrendous smell was still lingering in the air, and there were patients in all of the beds, bar one. Suddenly, a nurse walked round the ward and closed everybody's curtains. Without realising, after shutting mine, she moved on to the next bed before closing them completely. She left a small gap, and I watched as four nurses moved the pool table, which was in the centre of the ward, closer to the beds on the opposite side from me. Then I heard wheels on a trolley squeaking getting closer and closer as a door slammed open. Christ, I thought, they're bringing the lunch trolley back! I was just about to look back down at my laptop, when a large silver box was pushed through the ward by two men, and it was followed by Adam's mum. She had her head in her hands as a nurse had an arm around her to comfort her. "Oh God" I cried, "he's gone! he's gone, mum!" I guess we all knew it was coming, but still none of us could quite believe his time had come. Nobody spoke much the rest of the day. The ward was quiet, it was sad and empty. And that feeling of guilt came screaming back to me. No matter how hard I had tried to distance myself from the others, no matter how much I had tried to protect myself from the pain and anger of another teenager being taken away, I still wanted to punch someone. I wanted to scream and shout and cry and fight. This just wasn't fair. It wasn't fair.

Thorns Amongst A Bed of Roses

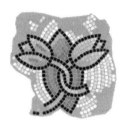

Despite the nightmare I was living at the hospital, and the heartbreak of watching others lose their battle, I tried to retain some sort of normality by going to school as often as I could. Walking into the Common Room that morning took all the strength and dignity I could find. I wanted to show these girls the reality of what I, and the other teens on the ward were going through, as I hadn't really heard from any of my friends since my treatment began. They had all really let me down, they ignored my calls, they never came round to the house, and I wanted to know why. Why, when other patients had cards and visits from their friends at school and from home, I had no one, not even a phone call. So I walked through the door with a façade of pure confidence, without Jemima, or a scarf and I was greeted by a deafening silence. Everybody stopped talking, stopped gossiping, stopped eating, they were all staring at me. Some of them even let out an impulse snigger. Lucy stood up, with her mouth wide open, staring at the top of my head, then she stammered what sounded like 'hello'. I asked her to step outside with me so she could explain where she had been for the last six months, at a time when I needed my best friend. I said I understood that it might have been uncomfortable for her and the rest of the girls to ask me to go shopping, or to the cinema, but she was supposed to be my closest support. She should have come round and sat with me, held my hand when I was in pain, when I needed a friendly face, but she let me down, just when I needed her most. I was calm; I simply wanted to know why she chose to stay away. I thought I had prepared myself for all her possible excuses; I had prepared a response to anything she may have thrown at me. What she actually said, however, I just didn't see coming. She looked me squarely in the eye, and said the reason she stayed away was because she thought she was going to catch it from me. I thought she was joking, "Please tell me you're not being serious", I replied, she said nothing. Instead she cried to one of our teachers who was acting as our Head of Year at the time. The teacher promptly called me into her office and asked me why had I upset Lucy? What had I achieved from upsetting her? I was fuming. I was right in the middle of six months of hell, and yet here I was being reprimanded for upsetting someone who should have been, but failed to be, by my side throughout it all. I was stunned, completely speechless as I stood in the small office. The Head of Year told me to put it behind me, that I was going to need all the friends I could get when I came back to school properly. She told me that I should be more considerate, I should understand that it was very difficult having a friend that was so ill. I'll tell you honestly, I have never felt so isolated or so angry. Inside I was screaming. What about me? Why shouldn't she have been more considerate towards me? Why couldn't anyone see how difficult things were for me? I'd only been at school for 10 minutes that day, but I walked out, and went home.

I tried so hard to carry on as normal. Now that I had Jemima, I felt I could go out and face the world, and try and do the normal things teenagers do. There were a few girls from school outside of my original group that would invite me out sometimes when they went shopping, or to the cinema. I find it very difficult looking back on those times, as after my treatment these girls stopped talking to me, refused to even acknowledge me in the Common Room. I couldn't understand it, it sounds awful, but often I think they only wanted to be my friend because it looked good for them. Taking pity on the girl with cancer, the girl with no friends, no life. I thought I had made friends *for* life with these girls, as they seemed to be there when I most needed support. But on reflection I realise that they too never came to visit me in hospital, they never came round to the house when I was feeling low. Only when it suited them was I invited out. How funny that the girls I had been friends with for years and thought would support me disappeared, and yet, when I thought I had found a new bunch of nice reliable mates, they let me down as well. When I look back I can see just how lonely I was, not really knowing who to turn to, who I could depend on for a bit of faithful friendship. Nevertheless I tried hard to look my best when I was invited to go to places with this new group of girls, I just wanted so desperately to be normal. I'd sit for hours with Jemima on her stand brushing her and trying to clip the hair back into different styles. It would be so difficult as often you could see the netting beneath, and I'd have to start all over again. Sometimes she'd look great on her stand, but as soon as I put her on my head, you could see the netting, or she wasn't sitting right, or there were little bits of hair sticking up and out. So I'd take her off, and start again. Mum would sit with me as the time would pass, holding Jemima's fringe so that she stayed still on her stand, as I sat styling the hair before taking it out, then I'd have to style it again, then take I'd it out, countless times. Never once did mum lose patience with me, although I would quickly lose patience with myself, nor did she ever complain that she had better things to be getting on with, and never did she tell me to just put a scarf on if she could see I was making myself late. I was always so paranoid people would be able to tell Jemima wasn't my real hair, so every strand had to be perfectly in place before I could even consider leaving the house. Like most things to do with cancer, Jemima and I had our good days, but we also had our bad. I remember one evening I was going out for dinner with the rest of the family. As normal, I had spent ages over Jemima with mum's help, and was finally happy with the way she looked. Just as we were leaving the house, I put my coat on and asked mum to comb the back of her, to make sure that she was sitting straight. Mum maintains it's because Jemima always looked so convincing when she was on, but as she brushed the hair she forgot to hold the top of my head, so poor Jemima went tumbling to the ground. We both stood staring at the rat on the floor, and burst out laughing. That day was a good day, and so I went out wearing my scarf. But there were other times when something like this would have resulted in me refusing to leave the house. The fact I couldn't just whip my hair up into a pony tail and leave the house in five minutes would often really get me down. There were many times I would stay at home and miss out on family meals or trips to the cinema because I felt so hideous, and Jemima was refusing to co-operate. How my mum didn't laugh when she'd walk into the room and hair would fly past her face from me throwing it in a temper. I lost count the amount of times I told mum to throw her away, saying she looked stupid on my head anyway. I'm grateful she didn't, as there were other days Jemima kept me sane, allowed me go out and feel normal for a while. Often at night I would dream so vividly that I had long hair again. In the dream my hair would grow really quickly, and I would run my hands through it delighted that I never had to fuss over a bit of hair on a stand anymore; excited that I had eyebrows, and eyelashes to make-up with mascara. I had these dreams many times, and after each I would wake up quickly immediately putting my hand to my head. My heart sank each time as my hand touched bare skin, the tears would stream down my face as I could see my shadow on the bedroom wall, with the outline of a bald, ugly head. And each time I lay back on my pillow and cried myself to sleep.

I started to have nightmares and hallucinations quite frequently by this point. It was hard drifting off to sleep sometimes, unless I was on treatment when I couldn't keep my eyes open, it was very hard for me to relax. Every time I shut my eyes I could see things coming towards me in the dark. I would jump and squirm in bed thinking that things were attacking my face. Thoughts would rush around and around in my head, crazy thoughts about dying and about my family dying, which would lead me to have nightmares. One night I dreamt mum, Dominic and I were attached to rockets. It was a very brief scene, we had been accused of something we weren't guilty of, but the authorities made us line up next to each other, with Dominic in the middle, and they tied rockets to our backs. We were to be shot into space, and of course would die as we travelled further towards the stratosphere. But my rocket was slower than mum's and Dominic's so I saw them explode in front of me. I heard them scream 'I love you' before they both broke up into tiny pieces. Then I felt my own body bursting, I screamed as I woke up relieved to find myself in bed, in one piece. But I was not always as fortunate as this.

Often I would wake up from a nightmare and it would continue as a hallucination, just as the doctor in Queen Mary's had warned me the night after my hallucination of the planes attacking our house. I remember one night, dreaming I was Saint Cecilia. My brother and I have been brought up as practising Catholics, and at 13 I made my Confirmation, taking on an additional name to mark a commitment to the faith, and usually, you would choose a saint's name, one that meant something special to you. I loved music at the time, as this was before my awful music teacher at school beat any enjoyment I got from it out of me, I chose the name Cecilia, after Saint Cecilia the patron saint of music. But I dreamt I was being executed as she had been. History books tell us that after an unsuccessful attempt to kill her by smothering her with steam, she was to be executed by beheading. They tried three times to chop her head off, but it didn't work, so she was left in agony for three days before she eventually died. I dreamt I was on a platform in front of many people waiting for the blade to come down on the back of my neck, then I woke up. As I sat up in bed I could see the shadow of an axe on the wall in front of me, it lifted up and I watched as it swung back down. I jumped out of the bed and screamed as I felt the force of the axe cut at the base of my head, and mum came rushing in.

"They're killing me!" I screamed at her, "my head!"

"It's ok honey", she said grabbing my face and remembering the doctor's advice to go along with what I thought I could see, "I won't let them kill you, they'll all go away now and your head can heal". She didn't have a clue what I could see, or what I thought was going on but she rocked me back to sleep telling me that she could see my head was healing. When I told her the following morning what I had thought was happening, she was horrified. I still can't get over how real those images seemed, even today I can see the shadow of the axe on the wall, as if it really happened just yesterday. I realised later that day, that this particular nightmare must have stemmed from the fact that the week before we attended my brother's confirmation. Perhaps in the back of my head I had been thinking about my own, and so the life of Saint Cecilia and her death must have sat in my subconscious until it came out in the most horrific nightmare that night. It's frightening to think what the mind is capable of, what it can make you believe, how you can feel so trapped in your own thoughts. It made me terrified to go to sleep, I tried so hard to think of nice things before I drifted off to try to prevent myself from having more nightmares, but it was impossible, they never went away.

In the meantime, I tried hard to keep up with my schoolwork, but it wasn't easy. I missed so many classes either being in the Middlesex for chemo, or in Queen Mary's having treatment for infections, and when I was at school, it was almost impossible to concentrate on anything. My mind would wander and I'd think about everything and anything other than what I should have been learning about. My arms would tire very quickly, The chemo was making my joints very weak and I struggled to write all my notes down, so I often had huge chunks of information missing. But I was trying my hardest. I hadn't had a history class for a while, so was excited when I managed to make it in for a class one Monday morning. I had my scarf on that day, Jemima and I had had a battle before I left for school, and I decided she should stay at home, it was so rare that I managed to get into school that I didn't want her to make me late. I sat with my new friends in the Common Room that morning, I had brought my lunch with me in case I couldn't manage the canteen's offerings, and put it in the communal fridge. Lucy ignored me as I walked past her towards the kitchen area, she had become very good at that, out of sight out of mind they say, but I still hurt every time she looked at me then quickly looked away as if she hadn't seen me. But whatever, I was having a good day which was rare, so I wasn't going to let her spoil it for me. As the bell for our first lesson rang I made my way to the history lesson, I was a little early, but I wanted to show I was still keen and wanted to learn. I had my folder with me, with all the notes I had written in the hospital bed since the last time I managed to get into school, and I had with me as much of the homework as I had managed to complete. I sat waiting for a while as the classroom filled, and eventually the teacher walked in. She was new and young, and very full of herself. I had only been in one of her classes before, so didn't really know her. She said hello to everyone as she walked in, and put her bag on the floor beside her chair. From her bag she pulled out a register and a pen and started to call out names from the list. She read a few out before she got to mine, as it was my turn to respond she said "Natasha, no? Didn't think so, absent again". I couldn't believe it!

"Actually, I'm here", I called out, and her eyes shot over at where the tiny voice had come from, looking stunned.

"Oh, I, I'm sorry", she stammered, "it's just you've been absent so much lately, I just assumed", and she carried on reading the names. I wish I'd had the strength to stand up for myself that day, to speak up, but I lost my voice completely. Why didn't I say, 'Yes, I've been absent! I have cancer! I worked so hard to be here today, to get here for your lesson, do you know how that feels? To wake up and start battling with a piece of hair so it sits right on your head, so that no one laughs, or to shower with a tube hanging out of you trying not to get it wet, to hold my head up high when none of my friends want to know me anymore?' But I didn't, I sat staring at the table, my cheeks blushing as I swallowed the lump in the back of my throat.

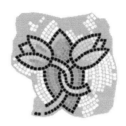

Life was a real battle during these months, in the hospital and out of it. But I kept going, spurred on by the thought that each cycle I got through was another one finished and over with, another one survived, and one step closer to the end. It was a battle each time I was due to be admitted for another batch of treatment. I struggled to motivate myself to get my things together and be ready for another week on the ward. The thought of being trapped, and tied to a drip by my bed was torturous, and with each cycle that went by, the more I dreaded going in. I was sitting in my grandad's front room one morning, mum and nan were busy loading the car with bags, pillows and DVDs. I picked up my bag full of medication and stared at it. Other girls my age carried their lives in their handbags, their purses, make-up and mirrors, and here was my life, boxes of pills, syringes and mouthwash in a clear plastic bag.

"You ready?" grandad asked.

"I don't want to go, grandad", I looked at him, our eyes glistening with tears, "please don't make me".

"I won't make you do anything, Natasha". I smiled and wiped a tear off my cheek. He looked so sad, I knew if he could take it all away from me, he would, in a heartbeat.

"Come on then" I said after a few moments, picking up the bag and walking through the kitchen, taking a little packet of white chocolate buttons from the fridge as I went, "can we stop off at the bakers for a sausage roll on the way?"

"Course we can!" Grandad replied.

After my bad experience on the train the first time I came out of hospital after treatment, mum arranged for hospital transport to take us home after the second batch of chemo. It was pretty convenient, as the nurses on the unit would call down and tell them when we were likely to be discharged, and a car would be waiting for us. The drivers were always helpful and so friendly, but we only used the service a couple of times. They were always keen to have a chat, so on the way to the hospital at the beginning of the week, and later when it was time to go home, they would always take their time, and we'd find ourselves enjoying a scenic route round the back streets of London to either destination. It took us twice as long to do the journeys and mum would sit with a puzzled look on her face as each time we took a different route. Now, this was fine on the way there, in fact, the longer it took to get there the better as far as I was concerned, but on the way back, it was an absolute nightmare. I would start to feel sick about ten minutes into the journey and we'd only be round the corner from the hospital! Of course, after a week full of fluids being pumped into me it wasn't long until I was absolutely dying to use the toilet. I would plead with them to hurry up—'nearly there love', they'd reply, but I'd have no idea where we were. Driving through all the little back streets, one road looked the same as the next, until eventually I saw a road sign I recognised, and I knew the loo was in sight! One evening when we arrived home from the Middlesex, grandad opened the door to us, "Where have you been?" He asked as the taxi pulled off, "you called to say you were coming home hours ago! Was the traffic bad?"

"No!" Mum replied struggling to get all our bags into the house as I dashed past and straight up to the loo, "the drivers tend to take us round the houses!"

"Well, which way did you go?" Grandad used to be a long-distance lorry driver, he would deliver beds around London, and all over England and Ireland, so he knew the streets of London like the back of his hand. As mum described as many of the roads she had recognised as she could, grandad burst out laughing, "that's insane!" He cried, "I could have got you back in under half the time! Right, from now on I'll be taking you to and from the hospital".

"Are you sure, dad? We don't always know when she's going to be discharged, there's a lot of hanging around waiting for doctors and pharmacy", mum said.

"Mary, it's no problem", he insisted, "give me a call in the morning when you're getting her stuff together to come home, and I'll try and judge it. I'll just wait outside in the car until you're ready to come out". So from then on, he drove us to and from the hospital every time I went in for treatment. There was absolutely nowhere to park around the hospital, it was on a main road with double yellow lines everywhere, and the only car park within five miles was tiny and for hospital staff only. But this did not deter my grandad from parking immediately outside the hospital doors. He'd usually get there a bit early and often had to wait for a couple of hours until I had been given all my medication and was ready to go, but he'd sit in the car right outside the hospital, only moving occasionally for the odd ambulance. On several occasions we came down from the ward ready to go home, and grandad would be mid-flow, screaming at the traffic warden who patrolled the main road and the hospital grounds, telling him not to give him a ticket, that he was picking up his sick granddaughter who was having chemo. I'd struggle to hide the giggles as we walked out of the main doors, and there was the unsuspecting 'yellow-cap' as he would call them, just doing his job, about to approach the car and grandad would clock him in the rear-view mirror. Now, my grandad was the nicest man you could ever meet, he would do anything for anyone, he'd put himself out by a mile if it meant he could do you a favour, he was lovely to everyone—except traffic wardens. After picking us up a few times and several run-ins with the traffic warden, the traffic warden left him alone, it was strange, suddenly he could park where he wanted, no one asked any questions, nobody gave any tickets. At times my grandad had a very special way with words!

We would shoot home at the speed of light, if there was any traffic, he knew a short cut, if any roads were blocked he knew a cut through, he'd keep us entertained with his country music and jokes, and before I knew it we'd be home and I could jump out, run to the loo and snuggle up in my own bed.

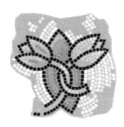

As my last chemo cycle approached I could hardly contain my excitement. I was like a child at Christmas as I realised that if the scans I had at the end of the week were clear, I wouldn't be coming back to the hospital for any more chemo, and the prospect of such freedom and normality made me almost burst with joy. Of course it was the longest week of all of them, each minute felt like an hour, each hour felt like a day, but I knew I was getting there. I just kept focusing on the fact that my hair would now be able to grow back, food would taste normal again, my body would have the chance to get stronger. I wouldn't need to come back to the Middlesex for three whole months, after which I would need a routine scan to check everything was still ok. I woke up on the final day of my final cycle and sat and waited patiently for Dr Whelan. After a few hours, he walked into my ward and straight over to my bed with a beaming smile, I could have jumped up and kissed him. He drew the curtains around my bed and turned to mum and I saying, "The scans you had last night are clear, we can see no evidence of any more disease, so there won't be any need for radiotherapy. Perhaps after three months, if there is spotting on your lungs, it may be something we will need to consider, but right now, you're free".

'Free'. After six months of a living hell, his words echoed in my head, but this time there was no sadness, no fear, no despair. I would never have to see another doctor, nurse, drip, or syringe ever again, well not for another few months at least, and I can't tell you how excited that made me feel. I still needed a saline feed for a few hours to help the last of the chemo pass through my body, and I longed for the end of the day to come. But I felt so guilty for doing so when two new patients were brought onto the ward that afternoon, they were right at the beginning of their treatment. I felt so terrible when my time came to say goodbye to everyone, with my little bag from pharmacy packed full of medication that I, hopefully, wouldn't be taking for much longer. As the nurses got excited for me and told me to get out of there, I felt awful, smiling and waving goodbye as the other patients looked up at me with envy in their eyes. Not only was I going home, but I was going home healthy, cured, clear, which was not always the case for everyone who left that ward for good. But I had done my time, and I just wanted to get on with my life now. As usual Grandad, nan and Dominic were waiting for us on a yellow line outside the Hospital's front doors, and we squeezed into the car for the final journey home. I felt so good, so free, as I wound down the window and felt the breeze against my face as we drove through London. I was expecting to have to go to Queen Mary's again the following week for one final treatment for an infection, but it never came. I didn't get ill at all after the last cycle, I needed no anitbiotics, and no blood transfusions, I didn't have any final nightmares or hallucinations, it was as if I stepped out of the Middlesex and the nightmare suddenly stopped. After a few weeks had passed I realised that now, other than having my Hickman Line removed it was definitely all over.

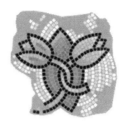

A while after I finished my treatment I realised I still hadn't had a period. They stop when you're on chemo, the medication makes this happen, but they normally start up again soon after your body adjusts to not having any more treatment. But a few months had passed and I still wasn't bleeding, I also started to get hot flushes. I could feel myself burning up and sweat would pump out of me, for no reason. When I felt myself getting hot, I'd take off as many layers of clothing as I could and stand in the garden. By this time, it was winter, and absolutely freezing, but I could have been standing out there naked for all the good it did, nothing cooled me down. I was coming up to having my first appointment being in remission, so I thought I'd ask Dr Whelan about it, just to be safe. I was nervous going back to see him for the first time since my nightmare had ended. What if he told me it had come back? That they had finished the chemo prematurely, and I needed to have more. I was just getting my life back, my freedom, I couldn't go through all that again. But mum was great as we travelled back to London on the train together, we talked about everything and anything other than cancer and chemo. The journey was quick, and soon we were sitting in the waiting room listening out for my name to be called. I didn't have to wait long. Dr Whelan called me through, and I was shaking as sat waiting to hear my results. He didn't waste any time, he could see how nervous I was, "You're fine, Natasha", he said smiling "your scans are clear, the chemo was a success, you're absolutely fine". I was so happy I could have kissed him.

"Thank you", I said to him, what else can you say to someone who has helped you fight such a battle?

"Now have you got any questions?" he asked.

"Well, there is one problem I'm having", I said, and I went on to explain the hot flush sensations I was getting, and the fact that I still hadn't had a period.

"Well, it sounds like the chemo might have brought on the menopause, Natasha".

"Come again?"

"I'm going to have to refer you to a specialist; sometimes this happens. Whenever a male is diagnosed, we recommend he deposit some sperm into a sperm bank as chemo causes infertility in men. But this is not always the case with women, and you're so young it was unlikely to be problem. But these symptoms don't look good, you really need to be checked".

"No, hang on a minute, I've gone through all of this treatment, a fucking nightmare six months, and now you're telling me there's more I have to deal with. Something that wouldn't be an issue if I hadn't had all this chemo! The fucking menopause! So you're saying I can't have children?"

"I don't know, Natasha, please try not to get upset".

"Upset? Are you trying to wind me up? I have to get out of here, mum". I got up and walked out. I sat on the floor in the corridor outside shaking even more than I had been going into the consultation. After a few minutes, mum followed me out, she pulled me up off the floor,

"It might be ok", she said, "it might be ok, and look, he just told me we don't need to come back for another six months, Natasha! Isn't that fantastic?"

"Yeah", I said, half smiling, "it is". Before she left the consultation room, Dr Whelan gave my mum the name of a specialist and said that he would make sure she got in touch with us over the next couple of days.

"I don't believe this", I said to mum on the way home, I was winding myself up, "how much more can I take? The whole point of being a woman, of being on this earth is to reproduce, to have a family. I want a family!" I was almost pleading with her. "Why didn't they freeze my eggs?", I asked, "they should have warned me about this, and I could have made a decision, why didn't they freeze my eggs?" Another thorn had presented itself on my rose.

A week later, we went to a different hospital, the Royal Free Hospital, in north west London, to see another doctor about my new problem. She didn't really have any answers for me, but said it was more of a waiting game, to see if my periods started by themselves. She suggested I take some Hormone Replacement Therapy or HRT tablets for a while, to help with the hot flushes, and she said that with time, the hormones in the medication may encourage my menstrual cycle to start up again by itself. So I took the HRT for the next six months. It calmed the flushes down immediately, it was great not having to leap up and undress on the way to the back door every hour or so, to cool off! Most importantly, as soon as I stopped taking the tablets six months later, my periods started again. I have never been so happy as when I got those first menstrual cramps and the back-ache that comes with it, to feel bloated with sore boobs and eating every thing in sight felt amazing!

Ending my treatment and returning to normal life was so strange. I felt vulnerable and a little frightened. Although, of course, I was absolutely delighted to be free, free from drips, and tubes and blood tests, and wards, and piss jugs and needles, and had danced out of the hospital the day my Hickman Line was removed. But I felt strangely unprotected, like I was now being left to fend for myself. What if I felt unwell? What if it came back? What if six months was too long to wait for my next scan, and the cancer got me before I had a chance to fight it? I had many fears and anxieties, I was so used to having a scan each time I was admitted for chemo, part of me wanted to keep this going, I wanted to go back for scans every few weeks to check things were ok. But another part of me never wanted to see the inside of that place ever again, and I began to appreciate the fact my life was no longer being dictated by hospital appointments and chemo cycles and infections. I very quickly got used to normal life, and went back to school full time. I wanted some normality straight away, but I was still feeling some of the effects from the chemo. Although I was now completely healthy, my immune system was still low, so I constantly had a cold for the first six months after my treatment. My joints were still so stiff, and my hair didn't start to grow back for a few months, so now despite the fact I was completely free of cancer, I still looked like a cancer patient, however, I was determined to get my life back on an even keel.

It was so much harder to get back into a normal life than I could ever have imagined. My taste buds soon returned to normal, chocolate lost that metallic edge, I craved foods that I hadn't been able to eat for months, so I ate, and ate and ate. My weight ballooned as I enjoyed all the foods I had missed so much over the past six months, but as my bones were still weak, I struggled to exercise to keep the weight off. Then there was my hair. It grew back a dull mousey brown colour, and I longed for the vibrant red it once was. It grew back like a baby's hair, soft, fine and really curly. I felt really patronised as people would say how 'cute' it looked, and felt they had the right to stroke my head to feel how soft it was. I refused to set foot in a hairdressers, I just wanted it to grow as quickly as possible, I didn't want to be trimming any of it off! But I should have, I should have styled it and looked after it, it would have grown quicker if I had, and would have given me a lot of confidence. I hated the way I looked with my silly short curly hair and my bulging waistline. And people can be so cruel. My uncle offered me some work experience with his IT firm in Holborn, he wanted me to grab hold of my independence and start working towards a future. I was slipping at school as I hated leaving the house looking the way I did, so he called me every morning for the two weeks I worked for him to make sure I was up and getting ready to get the train into London. It was nice to be travelling into London for something other than treatment and visits to hospitals, and as the days passed I started to really enjoy it. Although I hadn't been to a hairdressers, I bought products for my hair, to try to style it to make it look nice going into work, and for the first time in absolutely ages, I started to look after my appearance. I began to feel a little more confident, and enjoyed my new found freedom. Until one day I was walking back down the Strand towards Charing Cross station making my way home, when a man stopped me in the street, he laughed as he said, "I'm a hairdresser, who the fuck cut your hair? It looks shit!"

I just stopped and stared at him as he carried on laughing. I put my hand to my head and replied, "Actually, it's just growing back, I've recently had chemo and it all fell out". Why I felt I had to explain myself and justify having 'shitty' hair to him, I'll never know, and as he stood stuttering at me I turned and carried on walking towards the station. I fought so hard to hold back the tears all the way home, longing for the ground to swallow me, wondering if everybody else was laughing at me too.

I found it hard to get out of bed in the mornings, I was still so exhausted from all the treatment, plus, I could feel myself sinking into a depression. I knew that I had no real friends at school, I was fat, my hair looked ridiculous, I hated what this treatment had done to me, it had completely stripped away who I was. Back at school Mrs Hutchinson would call my mum in the mornings to see if I was coming in that day, sometimes, she would even come round to the house and take me in herself! It was very embarrassing pulling up at school in the head teacher's car, but I knew that she cared, and didn't want me to throw all my hard work away.

In the common room, I tried so hard to forgive and forget. I wanted to slip back into my original group of friends, pretend that nothing happened, that we were all as close as we used to be, friends forever. But I was too hurt, it wasn't the same, I knew I couldn't rely on them to be there for me when I really needed them, when it really mattered, and I couldn't afford to get close to them again, in case the disease returned and they let me down once more. Nevertheless, I knew that if I wanted a normal life, to go out to clubs and pubs etc, I had to make a bit of an effort, so I tried hard to get along with them all, including Lucy. Gradually, as my hair started to grow, and as I was able to exercise, my friends began to start speaking to me again, and so I got on with life. I managed to get a weekend job in a little pet store, just outside Sidcup in a town called Bexleyheath, and I absolutely loved it. I was the new girl so was always given the jobs no one else wanted to do which was usually cleaning out the puppy pens! The pens were always full of excitable little dogs, each of them a full-time poo machine, but after some of things I had seen and smelt at the hospital, it was nothing! I would be sent in every 15 minutes to clean them out, but I didn't mind. I loved having cuddles with all of them, they were always so happy to see me, so loveable! I wanted to take them all home! After a while, the shop was shut down, I'm still not sure why or what happened, but I soon found a new job, this time at the Disney Store in the Bluewater shopping centre, in Dartford. I could feel myself getting into a routine, earning myself a little bit of money, and I was enjoying my very first taste of independence. I started to look after myself again and decided it would be fun as well as fantastic exercise to learn how to belly-dance, soon the weight began to fall off. I started seeing boys, which was still a little alien to me, feeling attractive for the first time in so long took a while to get used to. I'd be in the pub with the rest of the group and a guy might show a bit of interest, I'd be convinced he was only talking to me because he felt sorry for me. With my short hair and awkwardness, I just couldn't understand what anyone would see in me. But I tried to get over this initial barrier of self-consciousness, and let myself go on a few dates with a couple of people. But I would always end up getting really frustrated, the boys I seemed to attract were always very ready to settle down and commit, and I just wasn't ready for any of that. I wanted to be free, and not have anyone to report back to. I felt I always had someone to answer to and account for my actions to, it wasn't the freedom I had dreamt of all those evenings sitting in my hospital bed. So I decided I was better off single for a while. Life got even better when I passed my driving test a few months later, I was slowly putting the nightmare behind me.

As the end of the school year approached, everyone was getting ready for exam time, but I had missed too much work. I took the difficult decision not to sit my exams and re-do the year in September, studying with people in the year below me. Of course the girls had something to say about this, they thought it was really sad that I would be moved down a year, they made me feel like a failure, they made me feel embarrassed. Little did I know that some of those younger people I was soon to be studying with would show such empathy and maturity, and turn out to be better friends than the girls in my year could ever hope to be.

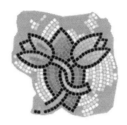

I was so nervous the first day back at school the following September, it almost felt like I was starting a new school, I felt eleven years old again. In fact I did consider moving schools, I wanted to be somewhere where no one knew who I was, what I had been through, no one could judge me. But my head teacher persuaded me to stay, saying that I had a good relationship with the teachers, I knew how the school worked, and besides, why should I let a couple of silly immature girls force me to move schools? I decided she was right. Because of the way the girls in my year had reacted when I told them I was moving to the year below I assumed the girls I would be studying with now would be just as bitchy. I had a little bit of knowledge on the subjects I had chosen from the year before, so I decided to just keep my head down, work hard, get my grades and get out of there. There were a couple of girls I shared my lessons with, one of whom was called Vicky. We became good friends, she was genuine and fun, and great to be around, and we remained close over the next two years, studying and going out together.

It was also around this time that Katharine, one of the girls from primary school got in touch. I hadn't really seen the girls from my childhood too much over the last five or so years, only in passing really, so I was excited when I got an invitation from Katharine to her 18th birthday party. On the invite it also stated that it was a reunion for our class at primary school, how she got in touch with everyone I don't know, but it was a fantastic night and I met up with all my old best friends, some of whom I hadn't seen since I was ten. As soon as we started chatting, it was as if we'd never lost touch, I told them about my treatment, and they were all so shocked but glad that I was healthy again, we all made a note of each other's phone numbers and we haven't left each other alone since! That was one of the best nights of my life, because I got my best friends back, Katharine, Louise, Rebecca, Justine and Emma, and through these, met more lovely girlfriends, true friends. They each helped me come out of my shell, nurtured my rose as the bud blossomed; they encouraged me to bloom. I now realised I didn't need those insincere girls in my year at school anymore, I didn't need to pretend I wasn't hurt by their ignorance, I didn't need to waste any more time pretending to be someone I wasn't. I had a brand new set of friends, for a brand new chapter in my life.

I carried on with my studies, and soon began to think about what my next step would be. I wanted to carry on studying, I wasn't sure whether I wanted a career in Law, Journalism or Politics, but knew that I really enjoyed all three. I was studying American History and American Politics at school at the time, and had fantastic teachers who encouraged me to stay on that track if I decided to go to university. Flicking through the University Prospectuses in the common room at lunchtimes, I was overwhelmed by the choice of courses, and the amount each varied from institution to institution. I worried about choosing one subject, and picking the wrong one, spending thousands of pounds on a course I ended up hating and subsequently failing. One afternoon, perhaps by fate, I was looking through Warwick University's prospectus, the grades were all so high, and I was worried I wouldn't be able to achieve them. Having taken a year out of school, I wasn't so confident now with my essay writing and exam skills, and I thought I was perhaps punching a little above my weight by even picking up Warwick's prospectus. I threw it down on the table in front of me in frustration, and I tried to grab it back quickly as it slid off the table. It landed on the floor upside down open at a page. As I picked it up, the top of the page read 'Comparative American Studies', and the description of the course that followed filled me with excitement. It involved courses in American History, Literature and Politics, and incorporated a compulsory year abroad in America. It stated in the third year of the four-year course all students were obliged to attend a university somewhere in The Americas, and it provided a list of Institutions to select from, including universities in the States, Canada, South America and the Caribbean. Sold! I knew then this was the course for me, and the Caribbean would be where I was headed. Curious about the course, I searched through the other university prospectuses lined up on the shelf in the common room, to see if any of them also offered American Studies, and to my surprise many of them did, some with the year abroad and some without. But none of them were as attractive as Warwick, none of the others offered the opportunity to travel to South America or the Caribbean, so I submitted an application immediately and crossed my fingers.

Mrs Hutchinson soon learned of my desire to go to Warwick, I spoke so excitedly about the course and what it had to offer, that she called the Course Director. Without me knowing, she spoke to him about my life over the last two years, she told him about my treatment and explained how impressed I was by the course. Soon after I received a letter from Warwick, offering me a 'Conditional Offer', this meant that I had a guaranteed place on the course on the condition I achieved certain grades, and they were two 'Bs' and a 'C'. I jumped with excitement as I opened the letter with mum, she was so happy for me, things were finally going my way. After overcoming so many hurdles, I had something exciting to work towards, I had a goal, and for the first time in a long time, I had ambition.

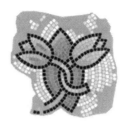

Every six months, when it's time to pick up my scan results from my consultant Dr Whelan I always make sure I book an appointment as late in the day as possible. That's because I know how the morning will go. I'll get up in plenty of time; have breakfast watch a bit of TV have a wash, maybe watch a bit more TV, get dressed, still glued to the TV. All the time I'm thinking about what Dr Whelan's going to say, tormenting myself with all the possible answers he may give me. I start to convince myself that I don't even want to go anyway, I'd rather not know whatever the results are, and I'll just live my life in blissful ignorance. Then I think to myself, well, everything's probably fine anyway, I'm just wasting a whole morning of my life to be told something I already knew. The thoughts go round and round in my head over and over, until I think I'm actually going mad. And so the time passes, and it gets later and later. Really, I should book myself an early appointment, the first of the morning and have it over and done with. I should force myself out of the house and up to London so early that I don't have time to mope around the house winding myself up.

The morning of 7th May 2004 was no different. It was two days before my 19th birthday, and I had an appointment with Dr Whelan at midday. My friend Francesca was due to come to the hospital with me, I arranged to meet her at the station and we were going to travel to the Middlesex together. It had been two and a half years since my last treatment, but even after almost three years in remission, I was no more confident about what the results would say as I was the first time I went back to see Dr Whelan after my chemo was completed. Of course, I was running late. I tried hard to be on time and not keep my friend waiting, but the usual thoughts played on my mind and stopped me from getting ready and dressed quickly. To get to my appointment in plenty of time, I should really leave the house an hour and a half before I'm due to be there, but at half past eleven I was only just running out of the house and down to Sidcup station. Before leaving I called Francesca and told her that I was running late, and I gave her a more realistic time to meet me by the ticket office, so I was surprised when I got there she was nowhere to be seen. I called her a few times but got no answer. Within a couple of minutes the train arrived at the station, and then left for the hospital with neither of us on it. I called her a few more times, getting more and more concerned for her. When the next train came along 20 minutes later I decided to get on it, I was already late enough. I was worrying about Francesca when half way to London I received a text message from her, simply saying, 'can't make it today, sorry, good luck'. Well, at least she's alive, I guess, I thought to myself, but it suddenly dawned on me that I hadn't been to the hospital to pick up scan results by myself before.

Sitting in the waiting room I started to shake, I was so nervous. I tried to read a magazine which was lying on a small table in front of me. I stared blankly at the pages as I flicked through them, trying to decide whether I was feeling sick, or whether I was just hungry, whether I had time to run to the loo, or whether I should wait to see if I would be called next. Suddenly I heard, "Oh my God! Natasha!" I looked up and saw a beautiful familiar face. It was Amy, a girl I had met a couple of years before. A little while after my chemo ended, a small charity in Scotland had been in touch with a few hospitals throughout the UK, asking if any of the patients who had been in remission for a while fancied a trip away for a few days to New York! It was a charity set up by a couple who had recently lost their daughter to cancer. They weren't rich, they didn't have loads of money to lavish on us, they were just regular, generous people who wanted to give sick teenagers the holiday of a lifetime. I had been so fortunate to be asked, I jumped at the chance. I had never been to New York before, and I had the time of my life celebrating my 17th birthday in a foreign city, with ten complete strangers, but with whom I shared so much. We would talk about our experiences, our feelings, how our friends reacted to us being ill, how we felt about moving on and dating boys, and we shared our thoughts about going back to school or work, and generally trying to get our lives back on track. This is how I met Amy; rather than meeting across a ward feeling sick and low, we shared a very happy time together. I heard that soon after our trip to New York, she had fallen very ill again, so I was so excited to see her that day looking so healthy, and with her hair growing through. She explained that she was at the hospital for her first clinic appointment in remission, she had finished six months of chemo three months previously and she said that she was feeling great. I was so happy for her, and she said that I was looking really well too. We sat together for a few minutes, and I asked her how she felt when she was diagnosed for the second time after our trip to America. She told me she already knew what the consultant was going to say to her. A few weeks before her diagnosis, she was blow-drying her hair and her arms began to ache as she was styling the front of it. After that, she noticed her arms aching a lot more each time she styled her hair, or held her arms up even for a short length of time. When she had her routine scans, they showed a large shadow present on her lungs, and her consultant confirmed what she had suspected. I took a bit of comfort from this; I felt fine, and had no reason to think anything was wrong. When my name was called over the Tannoy I jumped up, kissed Amy goodbye as she wished me luck, and confidently strode into the consultation room. As I closed the door behind me I was startled to see that it wasn't my Consultant Dr Whelan sitting behind the desk, but a young, tall, blond doctor with gorgeous big blue eyes. I stared at him with my mouth open as he shook my hand firmly and introduced himself as Dr Whelan's registrar, saying he hoped I didn't mind him seeing me today, as my normal doctor was rather busy.

"No, no", I stammered, "I don't mind at all!" I sat down, still gawping at him, and waited for him to smile and say everything was fine. He did smile as he asked if I had come alone. I started to ramble on about how my friend Francesca was supposed to have come with me but she didn't turn up at the station, but it's ok because I just saw another friend in the waiting room outside and I'm so relieved because she had been really unwell but now she's much better and is looking great, when he took hold of my hand.

"Natasha", he said, "we can see something on your kidney". I just sat and stared at him.

"No, I don't think so", I whispered, "you must be mistaken, I feel fine, I don't feel anything!" The registrar explained that I wouldn't necessarily be able to feel anything, they had caught it early, and that it was probably a good thing that I couldn't feel any pain, but that didn't make it any less serious. Everything seemed to go so fast. He called in a female nurse while he examined my breathing, and my ears, nose and throat, all the while my eyes were stinging. I couldn't cry, because I couldn't quite believe what was happening, but at the same time I wanted to scream and punch the wall. Just like throughout my first diagnosis, it felt like I was standing still while everyone else rushed around me, I couldn't take it in. As I lay on the bed with the registrar tapping on my chest, my stomach sank as I thought, how the fuck am I going to tell my mum?

I left the consultation room with the registrar's words still ringing in my ears. He said that he would be in touch later in the week to inform me when my follow up scans would be to check that the rest of my body was clear, and when my Hickman Line would be inserted. Christ, I thought, this *is* really happening. I was right in the middle of my A levels, I couldn't understand why this disease was so intent on ruining my hopes of a good career, and a successful life. Angry, I left the hospital in a sort of dream, trying to work out how I was going to break the news to mum. I decided to wait and tell her when I got home, rather than telling her over the phone, I wanted to be with her for a cuddle when I heard myself saying it out loud, so I picked up my pace and headed for the tube station. Just as I approached the entrance, my phone rang, it was mum. I didn't want to ignore the call and have her worry about me so I answered it. "How did you get on?" She said straight away.

"Er, yeah, everything's fine mum", I lied, the words just sort of fell out of my mouth. I just couldn't bring myself to tell her on the phone, and I wasn't yet ready to admit it to myself.

"Great! You clever girl! Get home so I can give you a big hug!" I never lie to mum, there's no point really, she can see right through me and always knows when I'm holding something back from her. But this time she didn't, and it broke my heart to hear the relief and delight in her voice when I knew in an hour's time I was going to take it all away from her. I got on the train, and gave myself time to digest everything the registrar had said. More treatment, more chemo, possibly an operation. I stared out of the window and thought, is this it for me? Is this just another hiccup, or am I going to have to live with this for the rest of my life? This cloud may never lift, this disease might just get the better of me. Is this a fight I have the energy to win this time? Or has my rose succumbed to the poison ivy that seems intent on wrapping itself around my bud? I was so lost in my thoughts that I nearly missed my stop. I took a slow walk home from Sidcup station, going over and over in my head how I was going to break the news to mum, especially now that I had made it even more difficult for myself by telling her everything was ok. As I put the key in the door I took a deep breath. My mum and aunt were sitting in the front room having a cup of tea, they were smiling and chatting, and their faces lit up even more when they saw me. Mum got up to greet me, "My little honey! Will you have a cup of tea?"

"Sit down mum", I said, I couldn't let her go on, "the scan wasn't clear", I gushed, "it has come back in my kidney, I need more chemo, I need an operation. We've got to do it all again mum!" She stared at me in disbelief.

"Are you joking?" she asked calmly,

"No, of course I'm not", I said.

"Well then why did you tell me you were clear? Why didn't you tell me?" She seemed so angry with me and it broke my heart. I explained that I didn't want to tell her over the phone, then make her wait an hour for me to get home, I said she would have been devastated and I didn't think that there was anyone around to comfort her. She hit the roof when she discovered that my friend hadn't turned up at the station, and I had been on my own. "Why didn't you call me?" she asked over and over again. She told me I should have told her I was going by myself, she could have met me there, I didn't have to be on my own. The funny thing was, on reflection it hadn't really bothered me that I had been alone. Without realising, I'd had a chance to digest it myself, and reflect on what was to come without having to worry about how anyone else was feeling, or try to comfort them as I had done with my nan on the train home the first time round. I was able to tell mum in my own words, and it somehow made it feel a bit more real. Telling my grandad that it was back was even harder. I called him and told him I was going to need more treatment, before I could even explain what or where the tumour was he hung up the phone and he and my nan drove straight round to our house. He arrived about ten minutes later and stood in our front room just looking at my mum, as if to say, 'Do something!' He just kept saying, "I don't understand, I don't understand". I told him what the registrar had said, that it was the same type of cancer in my right kidney, that I would need more chemo, probably for around six months again, and if it was successful, they would probably remove the kidney at the end of the treatment to prevent further problems.

"So why don't they just operate now, without having any more chemo, rather than you having to go through all those infections again?" he asked. I explained as best I could that it was to reduce the size of the tumour, so it is safer to remove the kidney, and also, it would help kill off any tiny cancerous cells which may be missed on the scans.

"I guess it's better to be completely safe, grandad", I explained, "rather than miss something tiny, and have to deal with it again in a couple of months". Then the tears rolled down his face again. He was such a wise man, bursting with knowledge and always full of answers, but here he stood in front of me looking utterly helpless, wanting to take it away but just not knowing how.

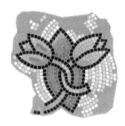

A few days later, I was still trying to come to terms with this latest news, when I received a call from the activities co-ordinator on the Teenage Cancer Trust Unit at the Middlesex. She invited to make speech at a conference due to be held a couple of weeks later, which is regularly organised by the Teenage Cancer Trust. Called 'Find Your Sense Of Tumour', the aim of them is to bring together teenagers from all over the United Kingdom who have experienced, or are still going through the trauma of treatment. For days before the event I made attempt after attempt to write my piece, trying to make it funny, and a bit light-hearted. But each draft I wrote ended up being torn in two and thrown in the bin. The day before I was due to travel to Nottingham where the conference was being held, my speech was still unwritten. "Just write how you felt", mum said after I threatened to give up completely and not go at all! "Be the voice for all those who can't be there with you", she encouraged. So I agreed to give it one last shot. As I started writing the tears flowed, as I allowed myself to remember the horrors of the treatment, the nightmares, the operations, the pain, the fear. As the memories flowed I questioned whether I could go through it all again. I didn't feel that I had the strength of mind or of character to face losing my hair again, to face losing my friends. All that time I had spent fighting illnesses, infections, nightmares. For a while I had lost who I was, but then a thought struck me—was it worth backing out now if it meant I would lose my life?

So I wrote my speech. I wrote how I felt about being so young with such a terrifying disease, I wrote about how desperate I was when no one was listening to my cries for help. I told of the deep guilt I felt for surviving, when so many of my friends didn't. I wrote openly and honestly; no jokes just emotion. It was a speech encouraging strength and determination to overcome whatever the disease threw at us. When I finished it, I put my pen down, closed my pad and went to bed.

The next day I travelled to Nottingham with my mum and my friend Siobhan. When we arrived I arranged a time for mum to pick us up later in the day, and I walked into the conference hall with Siobhan. The atmosphere was so relaxed, and everybody was very welcoming. There were a few people scattered around that I recognised from my ward in the Middlesex, but they were amongst a sea of hundreds of teens that I didn't. I couldn't believe how many of us there were. Some were still on treatment, others bared the scars of the disease they had triumphed over, but many looked so healthy, you would never have been able to imagine the pain they had endured. We took our seats, I was on the front row, along with a few others who had come to tell their tales. I listened to their stories and fear and anger grew inside, over and over I heard how others just like myself pleaded with medics to recognise the pain they were in. One girl told of how she paid her GP tens of visits over two years, because of a pain she was suffering in her shoulder. Her story was all too familiar as she told of how her doctor turned her away time after time, always with stronger painkillers. When the pain refused to subside, her GP sent her to a physiotherapist who made her move her shoulder and circle her arms for hours each day despite the excruciating pain she was in. When she was finally given a scan of her arm, radiographers found a tumour the size of a melon; it had dislocated her shoulder blade. Just imagine the agony she must have been in while doing those exercises. Next a young man told his story, he focused on his stay in hospital and his feelings about chemotherapy and the effects it had on him. I started to panic about the treatment I was about to face yet again, I looked down at the sweaty piece of paper with my speech on it, and felt like a fraud. How could I stand up in front of hundreds of teenagers and tell them to be strong, to fight the battle to reach that light at the end of the tunnel, when all I could see myself was darkness. I beckoned over a Teenage Cancer Trust volunteer, and asked her to cut me from the programme. She looked at me and smiled. "People want to hear what you have to say, love", she said. I shook my head and looked down at my paper again. "Here, I'll read it for you," she suggested, "but I want you standing next to me as I do". I agreed, and suddenly my name was called. The two of us walked up the stairs at the side of the stage. The spotlight shone so brightly on my face, and as I heard my words being read, I looked around at the sea of faces. Each person sitting in the hall was silent, listening to every word of my story. Some were nodding and smiling, perhaps recognising experiences I had described as being similar to their own. As I listened to my words ring around the conference room, the feeling of being a fraud melted away, and was replaced by that of pride. I knew that if I could get through that nightmare once before, I could bloody well do it again. Only this time my eyes were wide open. As the lady from the Teenage Cancer Trust came to the end of the speech, the words, 'So you see, having cancer shouldn't fill you with fear, instead, it should make you stronger', lingered in the air for a few seconds. Suddenly, the silence was broken by a man as he shouted 'YES!' and he stood up clapping really loudly. He was immediately followed by the rest of the audience, and I felt so honoured as everybody who could stand up, did stand up, as they clapped and cheered me. That moment told me that I would be ok. Of course I was very aware that it wouldn't be easy, but with support from people and patients like the ones applauding and smiling back at me now, giving up simply wasn't an option. As I stood on the stage tingling, I felt humbled. How funny that I came here with the intention of inspiring others, telling them of a light that waited for them at the end of a very dark tunnel. When in reality it was all of those people in the audience that day, who picked *me* up, and guided *me* towards that light.

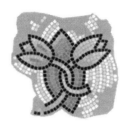

I worried about how my new set of friends would react to the news that I would need more treatment, whether I would lose friendships all over again. But I was so wrong, they were great. The few friends I had in school in my new year group, the friends I had made out of school, and the girls from primary school I had just started seeing again did not let me down. I had fantastic support, so different from the first time round. The girls from school and I had booked a holiday to the Algarve in Portugal before the exams had began, and we were due to fly out the day after our final A level. Dr Whelan said I could still go, and I would start my treatment as soon as I got back. So we made sure we had a brilliant few days in the sun. I knew what was waiting for me when I got home, so I relaxed and drank and danced as much as I could, and they were all right behind me, dancing with me.

I made the decision to have my head shaved this time. I hated the thought of waiting and waiting for it to fall out as I had done the first time round. So in between having my Hickman Line inserted and my first five days of chemo, I went to a small hairdressers and asked them to shave it off. It was a way for me to regain some sort of control over what was happening to my body. Of course, if I'd had my way it wouldn't be falling out at all, but this time I made sure I lost it when I was ready, when I was feeling strong enough. Luckily, I hadn't thrown Jemima away. She was in her box at the back of the cupboard in my room, and as I took her out and put her on her stand and combed her, I remembered the strength she gave me the last time. But my hair was a different colour now, it was much darker, and not red like Jemima was, so I decided another trip to Trendco was in order to update my look. The shop was exactly as I had remembered it, small, discreet and fabulous, and once again I left feeling beautiful, only this time with Chloe!

So I got ready for it to begin all over again, more treatment every three weeks, more infections, and another Hickman Line. I walked into the ward with my little suitcase wheeling behind me, one of the wheels was squeaking as it turned. This place hadn't changed a bit. As we walked through the double doors the smell of alcho-wipes, pee and lunch hit me, like a brick to the face. I walked up to the desk, and a familiar face looked up at me from a pile of paperwork. "Vincey!" It was Katie, one of the nurses, who had treated me during my first batch of chemo three years previously. She ran around the desk to give me a hug, then she turned back to the desk and picked up my heavy file, packed full of paperwork and information from the last nightmare. She pointed out which bed was to be mine for the rest of the week, then she took out a form from my file and began to ask me questions from it. As I gave her my full name, date of birth, address and so on, a single tear fell down my face. In a single second all my memories from my last lot of treatment came screaming back. The hallucinations,

my hair, my skin, my friends, all filled my head at once. I
thought my head was about explode. "How are you feeling
about being back?" was Katie's final question. My tears
answered her as I turned and walked over to my bed.

I was not as fortunate with my second Hickman Line
as I had been with my first. It was no one's fault, it just
happens that way sometimes. I had trouble with it from the
very start. It was constantly infected; either externally as it
came out of my skin, or internally—around and actually
inside the tube. I only had it in for about two months in
all, and hardly had any chemo through it as it was far too
dangerous. If the line is infected and fluids (saline, chemo
etc) are pushed through it, they can carry the infection into
your body, and so if the infection in the line isn't treated
and doesn't clear up it will keep making you ill. This is the
problem I had, the infection just wouldn't flush out of the
line, no matter how many antibiotics the doctors fed though
it. I had to have most of my chemo fed through a simple
drip inserted into the back of my hand, despite the fact that
carries its own risks, and they couldn't even take blood from
the line. Eventually, the doctors decided to take the line
out. I was on the Teenage Cancer Trust Unit, and supposed
to be having my next session of chemo, but my infected line
was making me too ill. I had a really high temperature and
was starting to hallucinate again.

The doctors agreed that the safest option was to just
get it out immediately, so late that evening a team of junior
surgeons came up to the ward to remove the line. I asked for
a general anaesthetic, I wanted to be put to sleep completely,
I really didn't want to feel the line being pulled out, I was
terrified of the pain. But the doctors refused, they told me
that I was too ill to be put to sleep. A general anaesthetic
would slow my heart rate down too much, and the doctor

explained that if I fell asleep, it would be very unlikely that I'd be able to wake up. They assured me that having a local anaesthetic instead would be much safer and they would give me enough to numb any feeling, they said I wouldn't feel a thing, and that it would all be over soon.

As they cleaned their hands and prepared their utensils, I lay back on my bed looking at mum. She held my hand as she reassured me "It will all be over soon, honey", she soothed "we'll get this manky line taken out, and you'll stop getting so ill. It will be so much better".

A nurse from the Teenage Cancer Trust Unit came over and put a line in the back of my hand so that the local anaesthetic could be fed through. I pleaded with him to ask the doctors one last time if I could have a general anaesthetic instead, "It's too dangerous love", he said, as he took my hand, "but let me know if you feel any discomfort and I'll feed a little bit more solution through".

"Ok", I answered, but I was shaking. Mum held my head away from the shoulder beneath which the Hickman Line was to be taken out. The doctor performing the surgery introduced herself and the rest of the team as the curtains around my bed were closed. She cut off the bottom two tubes that came out underneath my ribcage, so that she would be able to disconnect the top of the line from underneath the skin by my shoulder, and just pull it up and out of the vein. Then she started operating, and I could feel everything. I cried for them to put me to sleep. I was screaming as mum held my head and I could feel the whole of the inside of my chest being pulled up as the surgeon tugged at the line. The infection was so bad inside and outside the line, it had attached itself to the inside of my skin. The team tried for half an hour before having to call for a senior surgeon. He arrived immediately, ushered in by the nurses. I was sweating as I begged him for a general anaesthetic, but he looked at my heart monitor and said it was absolutely impossible. All the while, the nurse was adding more and more local anaesthetic, but it was doing nothing, it had absolutely no effect. The surgeon ordered more utensils up from his operating theatre downstairs, and a procedure that should have been completed in 20 minutes, was still being carried out two hours later. The nurse tried to take my mum away, it must have been so upsetting for her seeing me in so much pain for so long, but she wouldn't leave me. Afterwards, the other patients' parents told her that it was heartbreaking hearing me screaming from the other side of the curtains, as the medics tried desperately to help me. As I looked up at the nurse, begging him for more solution, I was struck by the helplessness in his eyes. He told me that now, he couldn't give me any more local anaesthetic, it was getting too dangerous. He put the syringe in a tray, and placed the tray on top of a cabinet beside my bed. He then took my hand in his, and rubbed the top of it with his thumb, then took my mum's hand in the other. I really wish I could remember his name to thank him. He showed such kindness—when he had done all he could medically and professionally, he could have just walked away and let the surgeons do their job, but he didn't, he sat and rubbed my hand.

After what felt like days, the surgeon put down the scalpel he was using to cut away at the infection and my skin. He then pulled the line out of my skin just below my shoulder, and the rest of the surgical team sighed in relief as the procedure came to an end. I was sweating, crying and in agony. I was completely exhausted, but so relieved it was over. I didn't even see the surgeon leave, I didn't get a chance to thank him or the rest of the doctors, I fell asleep, and didn't wake up until the following afternoon.

Before the Hickman was removed, the hospital tried hard to feed my chemo through, and administer treatment in the safest way. They were very patient as they waited for the infections to clear, but it meant I was in hospital for a month having this chemo cycle. Each time they fed the chemo through I started to hallucinate and show signs of an infection, so they'd stop for a few days, give me some antibiotics, then try again a few days later. It was awful being kept on the ward for such a long time. Every Friday night I'd sit looking out of my window, comparing the ward to a prison cell. I should have been out with my friends, I should have been drunk, I should have been dancing in the London clubs, falling out of taxis on the way home, I shouldn't have been here. Once again, I had been robbed of any fun, the normality of life, and the freedom of youth, by my illness.

One Friday evening, after two weeks of sitting staring at the walls, I'd had enough, I was 19 not 91 so I got my make-up bag out of the drawer beside my bed. I carried it around with me, but hardly ever applied it, I couldn't see the point. But today was different, I wanted to make myself feel pretty, glamorous, I wanted to be normal. I wanted to do what all my friends would have been doing at that time. So I opened the bag and spread my make-up all over the bed in front of me; my mascara, eye shadow, blusher, powder, and finally my mirror. I sat with my knees up on the mattress and balanced the mirror between them. Then I put on my eyeliner, carefully all around the top of my eyelids, and when that was done, I picked up my foundation, and began applying it to my cheeks and forehead. I laughed to myself as I noticed the huge colour contrast between the skin on my face, and my scalp, but I carried on, I didn't care. Just then, another patient's dad walked onto the ward. He was such a lovely man, he and his family hadn't been coming to the hospital long, and his little girl was dying. She had been brought in too late, so the treatment she was having was designed to subdue the pain and make her as comfortable as possible in the short time she had left. He wasn't bitter, he wasn't angry, not in front of us anyway, instead, he wanted to make her and the rest of us as happy and relaxed as possible. The first day they arrived, he made sure she was settled and comfortable, then he went to a florist down the road and bought all the patients flowers. Other than myself and his daughter, the rest of the teens on the ward that day were boys, so he bought them white roses, and he presented his daughter and myself with pink roses. "We need to brighten this place up a little don't you think?" he said, as he brought my bouquet over to my bed. Everyone was so touched, even a couple of the boys started to get a little emotional. But the nurses told him we couldn't have flowers on the ward, in case people were allergic, I watched as his face dropped. I hadn't had a bouquet of roses bought for me in quite some time, and I wanted mine to stay by my bed!

"What if none of us are allergic, can we keep them?" I called out. I looked around at the boys, as they each confirmed that they had no allergy and wanted the flowers to stay on the ward. The nurses looked at each other and rolled their eyes, laughing as they agreed we could have them, but pointed out that because it was the ward's policy not to have flowers, there were no vases to put them in. My mum jumped up and ran to the kitchen, two minutes later she brought back with her the biggest glasses she could find in the cupboards, filled them with water, and she and the lovely man handed them out to each patient, helping them put their bunch of flowers into each one.

He was very kind, very genuine, and able to lift your spirits in one simple sentence. As he walked past me putting my make up on that evening he smiled as he headed towards his daughter's bed. Just then, he stopped suddenly and turned back round to face me and called over, "You don't need any of that. You're beautiful".

He took his daughter home just a few days later, to be with the people who loved her when it was time to say goodbye, he took her away from the machines, the drips, the medication. The day after she left the ward, I noticed that the petals on my roses were withering, and some of them had fallen off and were lying on top of my bedside cabinet. I looked around the ward at the other beds and noticed that all the beautiful roses the man had bought us a few days previously were also dying—perhaps just as his beautiful rose was.

A few days later, we had a new girl on the ward. She was given her chemo in the form of a pill, so was only around for few hours as she waited for pharmacy to bring up her medication. She had been on treatment for a while, but her chemo was relatively mild, so she didn't have many of the side effects the rest of us had, and her hair wasn't going to fall out. She sat on a bed on the opposite side of the ward to me a couple of beds along. The rest of us sat doing our own thing, getting on with the usual routine, reading or sleeping or throwing up, when the new girl started shooting off her mouth. Surrounded by frail, sick teenagers with no hair she proclaimed at the top of her voice, "This chemo's a drag, having to come up here once a fortnight, but thank God I'm not as ill as this lot, and still have my hair", as she flicked her mane around her hands, and ruffled the back of it. Well, I don't know which us was about to knock her out first. If we hadn't all been tied to our drips and machines, she'd have been in serious trouble! But before she could even finish the sentence, one of the nurses jumped up and rushed over to her, telling her to leave it out as she drew the curtains around her bed. She wasn't brought back up to the ward after that incident, judging by the look on some of the patient's faces, it was probably safer that way!

One evening, it was really quiet on the ward. I was the only girl and the rest of the beds were occupied by boys. A couple of them felt well enough to play each other at pool on the table in the centre of the ward. I watched them for a while before dozing in and out of sleep. Suddenly my tummy started making awful noises, "Oh! I think I need to use the loo mum!" But as soon as I stood up I knew I couldn't get there in time, "I might need the commode", I whispered to her.

"Ok, I'm on it!" Mum said as she jumped up and quickly drew the curtains before she went to find a nurse. But it was too late, I felt so humiliated as I stood by the bed and could feel myself going to the toilet there and then. I had no control, and I stood looking at mum, tears streaming down my face. "Don't worry honey!" she said, as she came running back to me, "we'll clean it up, it's not your fault!"

"I'm sorry!" I said, "I'll do it, I just need a bucket of water, please".

"No honey, just stay there, I'll get something to clean you up with". I was mortified, I felt like an old lady, not able to control herself, watching as other people ran round cleaning up after me. I kept the curtains closed that night, I was too embarrassed to face the boys on the ward, not that they would have judged me, Christ knows, I saw enough of them piss and shit themselves, but it didn't make me feel any less humiliated. I felt so dirty and degraded, I just wanted to go home.

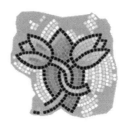

So the nightmare continued I lost my taste buds, was falling asleep all over the place and still couldn't cope with pissing in a jug! Midway through this batch of treatment, the hospital told me they wanted to take some of the stem cells from my blood stream. They needed to do this in order to preserve them and store them away, if I needed a transfusion of a particular type of cell later on in my treatment they would now be able to go to my little bank and retrieve whatever I needed. It sounded simple enough, they would need to take blood using a big machine for a couple of hours and they could do this via my Hickman Line. "I don't have that anymore", I said, looking at the specialist who had come to explain the procedure.

"Ok", she replied, "things might be a little more difficult in that case. We need to use a large, strong vein, one that's unlikely to collapse. What are the veins in your arms like?"

"Well, they're shattered, I've been having all my chemo through them because I don't have a Hickman, so the few

I have left collapse all the time", I said, thinking I had got out of it.

"Then I'm afraid we're going to have to use a vein in your groin, my love", was her solution.

"Come again?" I exclaimed! "Can I be put to sleep?" That had become my answer to everything now!

"No, that's not necessary. You'll be fine, the doctor does this procedure all the time, it'll be a little uncomfortable, but you're in good hands". Hmm, I thought to myself, 'uncomfortable', how many times had I been told that before?

"Ok, I guess" I replied as she arranged for the procedure to be carried out that afternoon.

"I'll come and meet you here on the ward before you're taken to have the cells extracted", she said as she stood up and walked away.

Later that day, a porter came with a wheelchair to bring me down to the basement where my stem cells would be collected, I thanked him but told him I could walk by myself, but he insisted I sat in it. I sat down, and took a pillow from my bed and placed it on my lap. I held it to my stomach, I had begun to feel really ill, but couldn't work out if it was the chemo, or nerves. A nurse greeted me as we approached the room in which the procedure would be carried out, and she wheeled me inside and over to a bed. Before I lay down, she told me to take my tracksuit bottoms and pants off, and handed me a paper towel to cover myself with.

"The doctor will need to get to the top of your inside leg, so you can keep this over your vagina" she said, so blunt and coarse. Christ! I thought feeling myself going red, I looked at mum as I took the towel from the nurse, she didn't know what to say. She held my hand to help me keep my balance as I got undressed, and lay on the bed with the tiny paper towel preserving my dignity. I lay there for a while shivering with the cold, and the nurse came over with a blanket, placing it around me from the waist up. Just then a male doctor walked in.

"Natasha?" he said.

"Yes, that's me", I laughed nervously, adjusting my paper towel, as he walked over and sat on a stool at the end of the bed.

He took an alcho-wipe from a tray on a cabinet beside the bed, which the nurse had prepared for him. Along with the wipes, there were blood bottles and large syringes with needles on the end.

"I hope my hands aren't too cold for you", was all he said, as he grabbed the paper towel, scrunched it up and threw it in a bin under the bed. I felt my heart thud as I lay on the bed completely exposed, my legs open with a man sitting directly in front of me. So much for preserving my dignity, this was undoubtedly my worst moment throughout the entire second lot of treatment. I lay in front of him for two hours like this, as he injected the top of my legs. I got a snippet of revenge though, and my God it was sweet. He was having difficulty finding a vein, it was so cold in the room which makes the veins retract, and from the pressure of the needle piercing my skin, my vein kept moving making it very difficult for the doctor to inject it, which meant at times he caught an artery instead. Each time he did this it caused a reflex and my leg shot up in the air, and yes, I kicked him straight in the face—did I feel bad? What do you think?

They thought I might need to have that procedure again once it was finished, my veins weren't really cooperating, and as a result, they didn't think they had collected enough cells.

Fortunately there was more than enough, I couldn't have gone through that again, it was so degrading, demoralising and mortifying, I think I would have had to say no, no more.

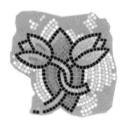

As the treatment progressed, the infections and other side effects manifested themselves again. I was brought into Queen Mary's hospital one evening by mum and Dominic with a high temperature and I had started hallucinating. This time the hallucinations were so bad and my mind was so confused that I no longer recognised mum and Dominic who were standing beside me. I lay in bed and could remember a life that now felt very distant. In my mind, I could see myself at work in the Disney Store, I knew that I had at some time achieved good GCSE results and was at some point studying for my A-levels, and I knew that once I had had a mum. But I couldn't understand how this life had ended. I felt trapped in my mind, and thought I could feel tumours growing rapidly inside me, expanding outwards and outwards as each second passed, I thought I was going to burst. I was so frightened. I struggled to sit up and tried to swing my legs off the side of the bed, but the lady I didn't recognise who was standing next to me kept telling me to relax, relax and lie down. She kept trying to force me back onto the bed, but I fought her off, I wanted to get up and snap myself out of this sort of mind lock I was in. I circled the bed, paced up and down the tiny room, opening and closing my fingers. I must have looked mad, and realise now how terrified my poor little brother must have been as he looked on. I knew I had to snap out of whatever trance I was in, but all I could hear myself saying was, 'I have to do something, I have to do something'. What I was trying to say was, I have to get myself back to normal, but at the same time, I didn't know what normal was. I was sweating, and crying, and in total mental disarray. My brother must have been petrified, but he stayed in the room with my mum, both of them trying to calm me down. Then a doctor walked in, he told me to lie on the bed. He asked me what my name was, I couldn't answer him, I didn't know it. He then asked me who the lady and the boy in the room were, and I told him I had absolutely no idea. But as I looked up at my brother who was holding a large heavy fan up to my face, I remember thinking he must be an angel. He had a glow around him, and was smiling at me. Thinking back logically, he was 'glowing' because he was standing in front of a window. He smiled in the hope that I would feel some recognition when I looked at him. But instead I just smiled back at the beautiful angel. I was frightened; trapped in my mind I knew something must be very wrong if I couldn't even remember my name. Just then grandad stepped into the room. I saw him so clearly; he stood wearing a maroon shirt with matching shoes and grey trousers. But he didn't come in to greet me, instead he called to my nan who remained outside, and told her they would come back later. I remember feeling really angry that he had just left me, surrounded by all these people I didn't know. The voices around me kept telling me to lie back and relax, 'just lie your head down and try to sleep', the lady kept saying, I was so exhausted I just did as she said. As I closed my eyes, instead of being plunged into darkness, it was as if a someone was shining a bright light onto my face. Suddenly I felt so relaxed, I was ready to let go. In that split second I remembered my mum, I remembered Dominic, I remembered my life and everyone in it. I felt no guilt about leaving them behind. I was so peaceful, for the first time in such a long time I was ready for sleep.

What felt like seconds later I awoke to the sound of a heart monitor, and could feel wires stuck to my body. A doctor stood over me as I opened my eyes and he was asking me what my name was, and if I knew where I was. I answered him, slightly confused at all the panic. Then I looked over at mum and Dominic and said "hello!" They both cried with relief, and they realised the infection was passing. As I began to recover mum explained that I had been asleep for hours, not seconds, and as I fell asleep my heart rate dropped dangerously low and they thought I was going to slip away. As mum reflected on what was possibly one of the most frightening times in her life, my own memory of what had been going on in my head over the last few hours returned. It was so vivid, and I explained to mum how frightened and confused I felt, how weird it was to be trapped in your own mind. Trying to snap yourself out of it, but not knowing how to, because you can no longer remember what normality is. I was terrified I would be trapped in that confused and very isolated state forever. She stroked my head and asked me why I had been looking over at the door for so long before I eventually fell asleep. I explained that I had seen grandad come in, and I told her how annoyed I was with him for not staying and helping me. She gave me a funny look saying that grandad hadn't been to visit me yet, in fact he had called to say that he would be up later that evening instead. But I was adamant, even now when I look back, I can still see him as clear as day,

"No mum, he was definitely here, he was the only one out of all of you I actually recognised!" I told her in detail exactly where he had been standing and what he had been wearing.

"I promise you", she returned, "he wasn't here". Funny, I thought, perhaps *he* was my angel.

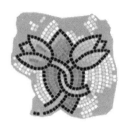

I think it's so important when you're having treatment for such a terrifying disease, over a long period of time, that you have a good relationship with your doctor. I trust my consultant Dr Whelan completely and hate having to see anyone else if he's unavailable. When I was in for treatment, now that I no longer had my Hickman Line, my veins would collapse all the time. The nurses had to be so careful that the chemo didn't poison me, that it started taking much longer to have the chemo administered than the standard five days. As a result I was often in hospital over the weekend, and the doctors on duty would be 'weekend staff' who weren't part of my consultant's team. I would get really impatient with them as they stood flicking through my two huge folders of medical notes, frantically trying to work out what treatment I was having, and where the disease was and what the next step would be. I always found them to be somewhat unsympathetic and unwilling to do or prescribe anything until they had received confirmation from my consultant the following Monday morning. Fair enough, but it always made me wonder why they bothered doing a ward round at all. I remember one weekend, I was having my saline feed during the day, but it was being pumped through too quickly. I was shuffling to the toilet literally every 15 minutes, and every time I went, the chemo from the night before burned a little bit more as it was passing through. There was so much fluid going through me, in the end I wasn't making it to the toilet in time, despite my bed being the nearest to the loo. The doctors were doing their rounds, and it felt like hours before it was my turn to be seen. As they stood at the end of my bed asking how I was, I started to cry. I told them how much pain I was in, I said that I was running to the toilet every quarter of an hour but couldn't get there in time. I said I couldn't take much more, I couldn't take the pain, I couldn't stand the humiliation as a nurse wiped the floor clean once again. "What would you like me to do?" One of the doctors responded. So I asked him to slow the feed down a little,

"I understand you can't stop it completely, but please, just slow it own a little, it burns when I pee, and each time I wipe it takes off a layer of skin". I was embarrassed, but I had to tell him, I needed him to understand, "and now, when I go, I'm not making it to the bathroom in time, it's too much, please slow it down".

"I can't do that", he said straight away, "I'm following instructions, and that's the speed it needs to be fed through at".

"But are you not a doctor?" I asked, "can you not make a decision yourself? You can see how I'm suffering".

"No can do!" He replied jovially, so I told him to piss off. I completely lost it.

"If you weren't going to do anything to help me, and you knew that before you even walked through the door, why did you bother coming in, why did you ask how I am, if you don't care? Go away and I'll see Dr Whelan on Monday, someone who isn't useless like you lot and actually knows how to do his job". I didn't see that doctor again! Some doctors have a fantastic bed-side manner, just like my consultant, while others have absolutely no idea—like the one I met that morning.

I was in my local hospital one evening, recovering from yet another infection, my hands were swollen from the chemo I'd had that week, and were so painful. A doctor came into my room to insert a canular. This is a small tube that is inserted into your vein and left there over short periods of time. They are used when doctors need to regularly take blood or give you medication, it's useful because it saves them having to inject you each time. A bit like a Hickman Line, but much more temporary and far less invasive! The one I had been using had started to come out, and needed to be replaced,

"What are your veins like?" he asked.

"Awful. I have my chemo fed into the back of my hand, they've all collapsed, and the ones in my arms aren't much better". As I spoke he picked up my right hand and started to slap and flick the back of it, I winced in pain and pulled my hand away. "That really hurts" I said, "my hands are really painful from the chemo, I've just told you".

"Well", he said, grabbing my hand again, "I need to find a vein don't I?" and started slapping my hand again. So I sat and cried in front of him as he carried on hitting my hand, still unable to find a vein, but he didn't care, at least that's how it felt. Eventually he found a vein at the top of my thumb, and as he inserted the needle scraped the bone. I yelped and winced again, I couldn't believe how insensitive this doctor was being, as he said impatiently, "can you stop moving".

"But you're really hurting me, you're really, really hurting me", I cried, trying to pull my hand away.

"Keep still please", he replied abruptly.

I could write another book about the shocking experiences I, and others I have spoken to have had with doctors, although most were great, and went out of their way to help, some didn't. It was just a 9 to 5 job for a few of them. It's not good enough really, it's all very well having qualifications, degrees and medical experience but if doctors can't talk to their patients, if they can't empathise with them, how can they expect patients to trust them? Or to feel comfortable putting their life in doctors' hands? You can't help someone get better when they dread the sight of you; it's a shame they don't seem to teach that at medical school.

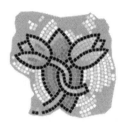

That summer, grandad took us all back to Somerset. It turned out to be the last time that we were all there, the five of us, and it was the best holiday I ever had with them. A fortnight in a little cottage was just what I needed in the middle of all my treatment, I had been looking forward it to since the beginning of the summer when grandad booked it. After so many infections and so much time in hospital, a couple a weeks relaxing by the sea was the best remedy I could have asked for. My treatment fell on the Monday morning we were due to go, and my A-level results came out exactly a week after. I wondered if I could ask my consultant to postpone the chemo for a couple of weeks so I could enjoy the holiday, but grandad wasn't keen on me waiting any longer than I had to, he wanted me to get the treatment over and done with. So that Monday he, my nan, Dominic and our little dog packed themselves off and headed for Somerset, while mum and I made our way to the Middlesex for another chemo cycle. Mum promised that the week would fly by, then we could pick up my results from school and head straight for Somerset the following

Monday. The time did pass quickly, probably because I was absolutely dreading getting my results. Having been diagnosed in the middle of such important exams, yet again, had knocked me. I worried that I had let my concentration slip, that I hadn't performed as well as I could have had the cancer stayed away and my scans been clear. I was terrified that I hadn't achieved the grades I needed in order to get a place at Warwick, I was angry that this disease had robbed me not only of my teenage years, but possibly the chance of a bright and successful future. I vowed, if I failed, to retake my exams once the treatment was over, I wasn't going to let this ruin my dream of going to university, I was looking forward so much to the course, to the year abroad, to the freedom and independence. "I'll do them again another time, when I'm better", I confirmed to mum as we walked into school that morning, "it'll be fine, I'll do them again", I kept repeating to myself. In the foyer a table had been set up and a couple of teachers were sorting through a box of envelopes, and as each student approached the table they were handed an envelope to open. As I reached the front of the queue, my head teacher called my name, I turned and she had my envelope in her hand.

"Here you are", she said, handing it to me.

"Is it bad Miss?" I asked.

"Open it", she said, walking away.

I needed two grade Bs and a grade C to secure my place at Warwick. I found a seat by the front door and opened the brown sealed envelope as mum stood beside me with her hand on my shoulder. As I read the Grades at the side of the page, I thought I was hallucinating again, 'A, A, B' it read, I couldn't believe it.

"Mum!" I screamed, "I did it! I fucking did it! Two As and a B! I'm in!" Mrs Hutchinson watched my exhilaration as I leapt up from the chair, holding onto my scarf so it didn't fall off in all the excitement.

"She did really well, didn't she?" she said, smiling at my mum as she walked over to us. I felt like I was walking on air, I was so happy, the chemo, the hospital, the fact I didn't have any hair, none of it mattered, I was so happy, the happiest I had been in such a long time, "before you rush off, there's a photographer here from the local paper, she's taking photos of all the girls with the highest grades. But I want you to have yours taken too, I'm so proud of you, I want you to be in the paper too, you deserve to be there with the rest of them".

"Oh, I don't know Miss, I haven't washed my hair!" I joked, she smirked and pushed me out of the front door onto the lawn by the entrance gate. The photographer was setting up, and she took my photo first. She didn't need to tell me to smile as I stood posing, my face lit up as I thought about what awaited me once all this treatment was over with. I had earned myself a future, something to look forward to, and work towards. She took a couple of shots, and afterwards I hugged Mrs Hutchinson goodbye as we got ready to join the rest of the family in Somerset for the remainder of the week. The car was packed and ready, and I sat holding my results the whole way there, still shocked at the grades staring back at me on the paper. What followed was the most fantastic, relaxed and contented week for the whole of my treatment. We stayed in a gorgeous little coastal cottage in Minehead, it had three floors, and my room was right at the top, by itself with a little ensuite bathroom. I woke up the following morning to the sun rising over the horizon. It lit up the whole room, it was so beautiful, and I could feel the sun shining on my face as a new day began. I decided it didn't matter how ill I felt, I was staying here for the rest of the week, there was absolutely no way I was giving this up to be trapped in a hospital. But I didn't get ill, I didn't catch an infection and didn't hallucinate. I did need a blood transfusion though, I was so tired all the time, and knew I needed blood, but tried so hard to fight it! Grandad would get upset seeing me struggle to keep my eyes open and kept nagging me to go to the local hospital for a transfusion. So I agreed, but only to receive blood, I didn't want to stay there any longer, and if I needed treatment it would have to wait until I was back in London the following week. So I went to the A&E department of the nearest hospital, which was in Taunton and explained that I was on chemo, was neutropenic and thought I needed a blood transfusion. All the staff were so lovely, they took a blood test which confirmed that my count was very low, and so I lay on a bed in their A&E department for a couple of hours as they fed blood through the back of my hand. One of the nurses came to me while the transfusion was going through to discuss the rest of my blood test results. She said my count was so low, I was likely to develop an infection within the next day or two, and suggested I stay overnight for a course of antibiotics in order to prevent getting really ill. I thought about it for a while, it might be worth a night in hospital if it meant I wouldn't spend the whole of the next week in hospital at home. But we had so much planned, grandad had an itinerary for each day we had left, and I didn't want to miss out on any of it. So I said no, and promised them I would have another blood test as soon as I returned to London to see if my blood count had improved. The rest of the week was brilliant, I felt relaxed and so positive about the future, getting those results and having such a lovely holiday was the boost I needed to crack on and get this nightmare over and done with. I returned home at the end of the week ready to face the rest of the treatment, determined not to let it get me down. Now that I had something to look forward to, a new exciting period of my life, and I couldn't wait.

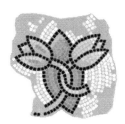

Once all six cycles of my chemo were complete, Dr Whelan booked me in for the operation to remove my kidney. The disease, from what they could see on my scans was gone, but he wanted to be absolutely sure there were no tiny cells lurking, and the only way to do this was to remove the whole kidney. I was terrified, for some reason I was absolutely convinced I wasn't going to wake up from the operation, I was much more fearful than I've ever been before prior to an operation. So much so, I wrote letters to people I didn't want to leave behind, my family, my friends, telling them how much I loved them. To this day I don't know why I was so terrified of that particular operation, perhaps it was because they were taking out a whole organ, but I knew it was my best option in the long run.

The operation was due to take place on the 8th December, I made my consultant promise, as we sat in his office, that I would be up and out and home for Christmas, "I can't see why not", he replied, "as long as everything goes to plan, and there are no complications, you'll be out in a week, guaranteed", he promised.

"Hmm, ok," I replied, "I guess it would be nice to have all this over and done with before Christmas, but If something does go wrong, you should know I'm not staying here on Christmas day, I'll discharge myself and come back Boxing day! There's no way I'm having turkey and Christmas pudding here! Ok?"

"Ok, Natasha, ok", he replied, smiling.

I had the operation on the morning of the 8th December as planned. They carried out the operation using key-hole surgery, which left no additional scars than the ones I had from my original operation. I woke up, and, apart from the pain, it was as though I hadn't been touched, it was incredible. I woke up in Intensive Care that evening. Because of the nature of the operation, the doctors had inserted a catheter, and given me medication to prevent me going to the toilet, so all I had to do all week was eat, and make sure I was up and out of there by Christmas eve. The nurses were lovely, always checking on me, making sure I was comfortable. They attached a morphine drip to the line in the back of my hand. It looked like a huge syringe, and they told me to press a little pump which was attached to it, every time I was in pain and wanted the drug administered. Well, as you can imagine, I was in pain all the time, and now I was in full control of my pain relief I thought I'd help myself out a little bit. I pumped away on the morphine, despite how itchy it was making me, until the agony in my back was a mild little niggle, then I fell asleep. When I woke up the unit was covered in Christmas decorations, and there were loads of cards and flowers and presents next to my bed. 'That's funny', I thought to myself, there weren't any decorations up when I fell asleep a few hours ago, and where had all those presents come from? How long had I been asleep? Seeing me open my eyes, mum jumped up and called over a nurse, "Honey", she whispered tearfully "would you like a drink?" and she brought over a carton of Ribena and placed the straw on my lips. She was so relieved, "Do you know what day it is?" she asked.

"Er, Tuesday?" I replied, very confused.

"It's Boxing day" she replied. WHAT? I had missed Christmas!

"Really?" I just looked at her.

"Yes, but you've had so many visitors, look at all the cards they brought you! And chocolates, you can eat them now that your taste buds are settling down". I couldn't believe it, I was so upset I didn't even look up at the cards to see them properly.

"What happened?" I asked her.

"You over-dosed on morphine, chicken, they've taken the pump away now because you can't be trusted! You've been asleep since the operation, you took too much".

I had done it to myself! I had made myself miss Christmas, the one thing I was looking forward to, now I had to wait a whole year again! I sat sulking for a while as mum nibbled away on the chocolates, after a couple of hours grandad came into view. Mum had called him to say I had woken up, so he brought nan and Dominic up to see me too. They walked in, so happy to see me awake, but I was still too traumatised, I just grunted back at them.

"What's the matter with her?" Grandad asked, "is she still in pain?"

"No", mum laughed before turning to me, "Natasha, I was just kidding earlier, it's not Boxing day".

"Eh?" Grandad grunted, "Boxing day?"

"It's only the 22nd December, you haven't missed Christmas", mum said laughing away to herself.

"Are you kidding?" I tried to yell at her.

"Well, I've been sitting here for over a week talking to myself, I had to entertain myself somehow, didn't I?"

"How mean is that?" I shouted over at Dominic, "can you believe she just did that to me?" But Dominic was in stitches.

"That's horrible mum", he agreed, but every one was laughing so much, I couldn't stay angry for long. I looked up at the cards which actually had 'Get Well Soon' and not 'Merry Christmas' written on the front of them.

"You're lucky I can't get up mum!" I smirked, "I'd better have a good Christmas present, that's all I'm going to say!"

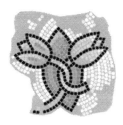

Soon, my hair started to grow back, I wondered what colour it would turn out to be this time. Each day was a tiny victory as my soft, fluffy baby fine mousey brown hair grew a tinsy bit more, but there were days it just wasn't growing quickly enough for me. I knew this time round I had to be a lot more sensible and less stubborn when it came to my hair. It would grow back much quicker and thicker if I had it cut regularly, and I knew it would really benefit from being shaved a couple of times while it was still very short, to give it a bit of strength and fullness. A new hairdressers had opened in Sidcup, while I was in the middle of my treatment, it was, and still is, a lovely little salon called 'Smudge', situated literally at the bottom of our road, mum had started to go there quite regularly to have her hair done. She always looked stunning when she returned, so I decided to pop along with her to one of her appointments to get some advice on how to help my hair grow a little bit faster. I hadn't been there before, I couldn't bring myself to go with my mum and watch other women have their hair styled, cut and pampered while I kept mine on a stand in the living room. The owner of Smudge, Debbie, agreed that it would be a good idea to cut my hair a couple of times to encourage a bit of growth, and offered to do it for me there and then. I hesitated, each millimetre of hair was so precious, but at the same time I knew that my hair would really benefit from this, so I agreed. Debbie was so compassionate as she shaved off the tiniest amount of hair from all over my head. She knew how important it was to me to have as much left as possible, and how patiently I had waited for it to start growing back. When she had finished, I could hardly see a difference, but the ends of it already felt sharper and healthier. As it really started to grow I had it shaved a couple more times, until a few months later, I was able to actually have it styled a little. I felt so glamorous sitting in the chair as Debbie suggested cutting it a little shorter at the back so that it looked heavier on the top. She also asked how I felt about having some colour put into it to lift it a little. I just looked at her, amazed that she was bothering so much over the tiny bit of hair I had. But I nodded in agreement as she pointed out a plum red on her colour chart, and she immediately ran towards the back of the salon to mix up the colour for me. What a difference it made, when she had finished cutting and colouring my hair I sat in front of a large mirror as she held up a smaller one behind me so that I could see the back of my head. I felt beautiful, as beautiful as a rose. Why hadn't I done this the first time round? I could feel myself getting angry, but it didn't last long. I was just glad I'd had the courage to do it now, after months of feeling so unattractive, I couldn't stop touching my hair and smiling to myself as I sat in front of the mirror with a beautiful reflection smiling back at me.

It was so nice to have a bit of colour to brighten my look a little, but also it meant that I could keep track of how quickly it was growing! Mum used to joke with me that I was the only girl she knew who was glad when her roots were showing. I'd sit and inspect the top of my hair every week to see how much it had grown, and pull it down over the top of my ears, laughing as it tickled, amazed at how quickly it was growing back this time round. I've been going to Smudge to have my hair done ever since, I wouldn't go anywhere else now. They showed such compassion and understanding when I was nervous about anyone touching my hair, I was so self-conscious, but in just one hour they changed my outlook completely. As I walked out of the salon with my newly styled and coloured hair I felt as though people were staring at me, just like I did when I lost my hair, only this time they were looking at me not because I was bald and ugly, but because I felt gorgeous and walked with confidence. I stepped out of the shop with my head held high, I felt so good you just can't imagine. How do you say thank you for a gift like that?

And so I started getting on with life again. I was due to start my course at Warwick the following September, so I had a good few months to relax, have fun and earn myself a little bit of money. I had a great few months, with no responsibilities, no hospital visits, no treatment. My hair was starting to grow back quickly, and to my relief my periods started again almost immediately this time round, with no hot flushes. But the cloud was always present, and there was always something reminding me that I was a little bit different, that my life wasn't as straightforward as most peoples. I started seeing a guy, I met him through a friend, and after a while I decided to go on the pill. I was taking blood pressure tablets at the time, to help out my one remaining kidney, and so I wasn't sure which type of contraceptive pill was safe to take along side it, whether one set of medication could cancel out or overpower the effects of the other one. I spoke to my local nurse, but she wasn't entirely sure herself and said it would be best if I spoke to Dr Whelan. So I emailed him asking him for some advice, he told me I should be fine to take any contraceptive pill with the blood pressure tablets I was on, but to keep an eye on any side effects. The next time I went to the Middlesex to pick up my routine scan results, I sat in front of him with my mum beside me as he asked how I was feeling, what I had been up to, and how I was getting on with the pill and the blood pressure tablets. I didn't need to look round at my mum, I could feel her face drop. She sat there silently as my consultant went through my scans, explaining that they were all clear, that I could live another six months chemo free, until it was time to come back again for another check up. I should have felt relieved, ecstatic, but I didn't, I felt embarrassed and awkward and I was angry that I couldn't just get on with my life without having to run everything past a doctor and my mum first. I wished I hadn't asked him about the possibilities of side effects, I wish I had just started taking the pill without consulting anyone. I was 20 years of age and yet I sat in that room feeling like a naughty little girl as my mum looked at me with such disappointment as she was forced to acknowledge that I was having sex!

"You're on the pill?" She asked, as we walked out of the room, I could feel my face burning, "why didn't you tell me?"

"Why should I mum? I'm a young woman, what I do is my business, I'm sorry you had to hear that, but please, let me live my life", I lashed out, mortified. But I could see she was hurt. After years of living in each other's pockets, and having to rely on her so often to do so much for me, I guess the thought of me breaking away and gaining some independence must have been quite hard for her. This situation reflected a difficult time for us, trying to readjust to some sort of normality and move on, but with mum still wanting to protect and shelter me. We clashed many times over the next few months, we argued when I stayed out late, we disagreed about my choice of boyfriends, we refused to compromise on anything. But perhaps this was all part of the process of getting back to normal, at least now we were arguing over things every parent disagrees with their children about, and of course, she usually turned out to be right anyway!

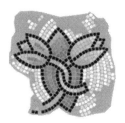

I continued having my check-ups every six months. I never got any better with my punctuality, each morning was exactly the same, panicking over what was going to be said, but each time I was elated at the news I was all clear. In the meantime I began my course at Warwick. It was a huge step for me. Having been living in my mum's pocket for so long now, moving two and a half hours away to live on my own surrounded by strangers was terrifying, for me and her. As I unpacked my life in my new little home, I got a bit upset as mum and grandad got ready to leave. "You just come home whenever you like, Natasha", grandad said as they left, "If you don't like it get in the car and come home, just like that".

"Thanks grandad", I laughed, as I opened my suitcase on the bed, "I'll be fine". But as I watched them leave I wondered why I was getting so upset, what was I frightened about? Having taken a year out in the middle of my A-levels, and again after them, I was now two years older than most of the people on my course, perhaps I was a little apprehensive about the reaction of my course mates, but this was what I had been waiting for for so long. I was staying in halls, so although I had my own room and bathroom, I shared a kitchen with a few other people, so decided to go and knock on the doors either side of me, to introduce myself to my new neighbours. It seemed everyone was just as quiet and unsure as I was, as there wasn't much conversation made when the doors were opened to me. But our warden had organised a drink in the Students' Union for us all later in the evening, as a way of getting to know everyone in a more relaxed environment. So I finished unpacking and started to get ready for the evening.

At the Students' Union later that day I met a girl who was on my course, Cat, it turned out she was staying in the room opposite me. I also met a guy called Andy who lived a couple of doors down from Cat. It was so strange when we got talking and realised we both lived in Sidcup, I even went to the same school as his sister! Despite being a couple of years older than Cat and Andy, we all really clicked and soon became inseparable. We had some great times that first year, and they were both so supportive and inquisitive when I eventually told them I had been ill, but they didn't treat me any differently because of it. I was really enjoying the course and had settled in completely as Christmas approached. I was on top of my work, and was looking forward to spending a few weeks at home with my family, I hadn't seen them in so long! As the end of term approached, I developed a really bad cold. Cat would stand staring at me in horror as I stood coughing and wheezing whilst we were on our way to lectures. "You know you really should see a doctor about that", she said.

"What? A cold? Behave yourself!" I used to laugh at her, "it'll pass in a few days". But two weeks later when mum and grandad came up to Warwick to help me move my things home for the holidays I was still so ill.

"Have you seen anyone about that?" Mum asked.

"No, but perhaps I should", I said to her. I was seeing Dr Whelan in a couple of weeks to pick up my next lot of scan results, so told mum if I was still bad, he could take a look at me then. But I was almost back to full health by the time I was due to go to the Middlesex, which, by now had become the University College Hospital which is adjacent to Warren Street tube station, I just had a little bit of the sniffles. As I sat in front of him yet again, my heart thudded as he put the printed image of my scan up against the light.

"I'm a little concerned about this shadow you have on your lungs here", he said. I started to panic, I could see the shadow without him having to point it out, it was huge. 'Fuck', I thought, not again, not now, I'm trying so hard to get on with things, don't take it away from me now. "It's either the disease" Dr Whelan continued, "or some sort of infection, I need to book a more detailed scan immediately in order to be able to narrow it down completely".

"Ok", I replied shaking, "I have had a really bad cold lately", I gushed, hopefully.

"Yes, well maybe that might be it, we'll see", he answered.

So he booked me a scan for a little later that day, with a follow up appointment a couple of days later. Cat was so upset when I told her, as were the rest of my lovely friends. "It might be nothing though", I tried to reassure them, as well as myself, "just an infection that can be treated with antibiotics". But I felt physically sick as I waited outside the consultation room a few days later to get the results of the scan. "I can't do it again", I said, turning to mum, just before we were called in, "I can't".

"Ok hun, ok", mum replied, as the consultant popped his head out of the room and beckoned me in. I sat in front of him ready for the worst, and he turned to me as he removed his glasses from his face, crossed his legs, and placed his hands on his lap.

"Natasha", he began, "you have pneumonia".

"Eh?" That wasn't what I was expecting at all!

"Yes, which normally would be really bad, but you seemed to have fought the worst of it off, all by yourself. You should have been in hospital for at least two months with this! But there's no point in me even giving you any penicillin now because your body has healed itself naturally. I'm not too sure what to say! You have a body of steel".

"Oh", I replied, not too sure what to say myself, "is that it then?"

"Yep, see you in six months!"

"Hang on", mum cut in, "are you sure? She doesn't need any medication at all?"

"No", he replied, it won't be of any use, her body has healed itself, and he held up my most recent scan which showed only a tiny shadow compared to what had shown up in the scan which had been carried out three weeks previously. He also showed me that it had left a small amount of scarring on my lungs. But that didn't bother me, it wasn't cancer, that was good enough for me! So I carried on at university, and enjoyed the rest of the year with my new friends. I worked hard, but played harder, it was the happiest time of my life up to then, I was so relieved that I had fought so hard to carry on with school and not let those silly girls put me off. I had given myself a chance to make a future for myself, but I was having a bloody good time along the way!

If You Were A Rose, I'd Pick You A Thousand Times Over

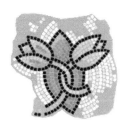

Then I met Andreas. It was the summer of 2006 and Cat and I were approaching the end of our first year of study at Warwick. Andreas was Cat's brother, Eamonn's, best friend, and during one weekend towards the end of the final term of the year he and Eamonn came up to Warwick for a night out. It wasn't the best of timing it being a week before exams, but Cat hadn't seen her brother in a while, and she was excited to spend some time with him. On the day they were due to come up, she called me at quarter to eight in the morning asking to borrow my straightening irons for her hair. The boys had just turned off the motorway at Warwick, and she was running around in the nuddy like a crazy trying to tidy the place up before they found our building. Unfortunately she wasn't quite quick enough; they blasted through the door shortly after eight in the morning, and our weekend began. Cat knocked on my door soon after the boys arrived to pick up the irons; I pulled myself out of bed and was almost blinded by the light as I opened the door to her and grunted something about the irons being in the drawer beside my bed. As she came into my room, I looked up and behind her was the tastiest bloke I had ever seen! Dressed in jeans, a crisp white shirt and navy blue blazer, he turned and smiled at me with a perfect set of teeth. He was tall, smart and gorgeous! As I closed the door in a daze I turned and caught a glimpse of myself in the full-length mirror on the wall. Holy Moses! It appeared that during the night I had crawled over to the electric socket situated underneath my desk, secured my hand in it, turned it on and held it there for several hours. It was the only explanation as to why my hair was pointing directly upwards towards the ceiling. In addition, having failed to remove my make-up the night before, my entire face had slid down towards my neck, and was now resting on my chin. I looked down and noticed that in my drunken state a few hours previously I had, fortunately, remembered to put on some pyjamas. Unfortunately, however, I had managed to pick out the ugliest, saggiest set I could find. Peach coloured, and very unsupportive. So there it was, I had succeeded in providing Andreas with the first impression of myself as a wolf woman-like saggy Morticia Adams, who had left her taste in bedroom attire, along with her dignity firmly at the door. And that is how I met Andreas.

We got on really well, and once my exams were out of the way, started to see each other regularly. When the time came for my first scan since we got together, I explained to him what I had been through before my time at university and he seemed to take everything in his stride. He asked if he could come with me to the appointment, and although I was a little apprehensive, I agreed. I was unsure, as up until now I had always brought mum with me to see Dr Whelan. She knew the procedure, she knew what to say, and she knew how I was feeling without me even telling her. Also I was unsure how he would react once we actually got to the hospital, whether he would freak out when he saw all the other patients in the waiting room, some with no hair, others with no arms or legs. But he had offered to come, so I thought I should at least respond positively to his thoughtfulness. As we got ready on the morning of my appointment, he tried his best to keep my mind off the day ahead. Even on the train to the hospital, he was larking about and trying to make me laugh, but I knew that deep down he was just as worried as I was. It must have been very difficult for him. I had become something of an expert at doing this journey by now, but for him it was all very new, and very daunting. We had only been together for six months at this point, and to be honest I was a little surprised at just how keen he was to come with me, but I appreciated the support. Perhaps he had convinced himself that I would be fine, after all, I looked fine, and I felt fine. But then again I felt fine the last time I was diagnosed. Sitting in the waiting room, he was winding me up no end. Slurping his tea, then he started slurping the soup he had bought from the vending machine, he was tapping his feet, and clicking his fingers, then he started to hum, a sort of cheery little tune. I was just about to smack him around the back of the head when my consultant's voice came booming over the Tannoy. 'Natasha Vince to room 13, please'. Room 13, was that a sign? I stood up, shaking. I was so startled, all my appointment slips, my scarf and my coat, my bottle of water fell and I stood watching them tumble to the ground. Andreas quickly scooped them all up for me, he grabbed my hand, squeezed it tight and led me down the corridor to my consultant's room.

I could feel my heart beating inside my chest, something was telling me that it wasn't going to be good news today. I wanted to turn around and run. As we were walking down the corridor I started my routine mental battle. I tried to convince myself that I'd rather not know the results, and that I was probably fine anyway, this was just another day wasted, getting stressed about nothing. I looked up and saw Dr Whelan waiting for me outside his office, no chance of running away now! He welcomed me into the room. I sat on the opposite side of his desk, with Andreas sitting next to me. He asked me the usual questions, How was I? What had I been up to since my last check up? I mumbled something about university and introduced Andreas. The doctor smiled, took his glasses off and put his pen down on his desk. "Your scan", he said. He didn't need to say any more.

"Not again", I was gutted. I was getting my life together, a career, a future. "How bad is it?" I asked. He explained that it had returned in my liver and showed me my scan. I could see three small white spots against a large grey shadow, which was my liver. I was so angry I was shaking. Andreas put his arm around me to comfort me, but I just wanted to scream. "This is never going to go away, is it?" I asked my consultant, I don't know what I was expecting him to say, but he just looked at me sympathetically as he began to explain the treatment he wanted me to undergo. A type of Radiotherapy called RFA, or Radio Frequency Ablation therapy was what he suggested. It involves a small operation to burn out the tumours from inside the body, rather than using radiation rays from outside the body as is usually the case with radiotherapy. It is an intense treatment, which can only be performed on the liver as it is the only organ that can actively repair itself. So, in many ways, I was very lucky it had returned there, and not elsewhere in my body. Otherwise, I would certainly have needed to undergo more painful chemotherapy. But as the consultant continued to explain what was to happen, his voice was getting quieter and quieter. Eventually it stopped, and there was anticipation hanging in the air as he awaited my response. "Whatever", I replied, "just call me when the operation is confirmed".

"I knew it", I said to Andreas as we walked back down the corridor towards the stairs, "I bloody knew it!" I fumed. But he just wrapped his arms around me, and whispered, 'I love you' in my ear. It was the first time he had said it to me, and just for a second everything around me disappeared. I looked at him, and I could see from the way he was looking at me he meant it. As we stood there another patient walked past, she was frail with no hair, gaunt and clinging on to someone who looked like she might have been her mum. As she staggered past, I asked "will you still love me if I need chemo and look like that girl?"

"Hmmm", he replied smiling, "maybe". He grabbed me, kissed the top of my head, then took me to a pub across the road from the hospital, and got me good and drunk!

As we took the long train ride home, and I was trying to work out how to tell my mum that we were going to have to go through it all over again, I sat looking at Andreas. I couldn't believe that this gorgeous fella, who I'd only been with for a few months, hadn't run away screaming by now! He seemed to be taking everything in his stride, and although I now know he confided deeply in his friends, he never once broke down in front of me. He was strong when I needed him to be, comforted me when I was feeling sorry for myself, but most importantly, was tough with me when I felt like giving up. He was everything I needed all wrapped up in a gorgeous package, my pillar of strength.

So I went ahead with the operation, and once again everything was sugar coated. Again, they told me that I'd simply be uncomfortable for a few days, when in reality I was in agony for three weeks. I couldn't eat, I couldn't go to the toilet, I couldn't walk, dress or wash. It was all just too painful. Over the following month, I slowly recovered. The road was bumpy, and I needed to go back into hospital several times for various different problems. The worst, I have to admit, was how difficult it was to go to the loo! With the pain from this, along with the pain from the operation, I think it's fair to say that I was feeling a little worse than merely 'uncomfortable'!

I took time out to recover, but returned to university a few weeks later, keen to show them that I was feeling better, stronger. I was in my second year now and was getting ready to spend a year abroad. I had chosen to go to the tiny Spanish-Caribbean island of Puerto Rico, and wanted to show my professors that I was ready and well enough to go.

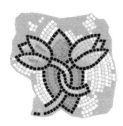

Sitting on the plane, a surge of excitement filled me; it was August 2007 and the beginning of the third year of my American studies course, which meant it was the start of my study year abroad in Puerto Rico. A year in the tropical Caribbean—my dream come true! I had been waiting so long for this. We began taxiing down the runway and I sat back and thought about all those months I had spent in hospital. Unable to go out and enjoy the sun, enjoy my freedom. I wanted to make the most of this year, to experience all the things my friends who hadn't made it were not fortunate enough to experience. But as we took off, the feeling of excitement turned into sadness and pain. Leaving Andreas behind was breaking my heart already, and I couldn't wait until I landed in New York to call him before our connecting flight. I had no idea how I was going to get through the next ten months not being able to see him, but I knew I was never going to get this opportunity again. So I tried to be positive, I had to go home for a scan at Christmas, so I knew I would see him then, and with the internet and phone calls, I told myself that the time would fly by.

Fly by it did. Cat and I landed at the airport in the Island's capital city Old San Juan, and as we walked out of the terminal the heat hit is immediately, everything was so different and so exciting. There were many gorgeous hotels surrounding the airport, and we couldn't wait to get to our accommodation, unpack and explore. We jumped in a taxi, and in our extremely poor Spanish attempted to inform the driver of our new address, which was directly opposite the main site of the university. It took us a while to make ourselves understood, there was much gesturing, pointing and giggling, but we got there in the end, and as we pulled away from the airport, I had a great feeling about our new life here.

After about ten minutes of travelling in the car, I noticed a giant tower block in the distance. It was getting closer and closer, taller and taller, and more noticeably dirty and dilapidated. I joked with Cat that knowing our luck, the taxi would pull up in front of the tower block and announce that we had arrived! "That's about right!" She said but then retracted it with, "no, no, Warwick would never do that to us!" Oh how we spoke too soon. The further we drove the closer we got to the huge building, we could see it was in terrible condition, dilapidated and in good need of a lick of paint! I couldn't believe it. As we pulled up outside and the driver turned round to us and laughed, Cat looked at me and said "Of course it is! Of course it is!" Called 'Torre Del Norte' or 'North Tower' it loomed over us. I was so tempted to tell the driver to take us back to the airport, I didn't know whether to laugh or cry! I had to keep reminding myself how much money I had just spent on flights to get there, forbidding myself from wasting any more by running straight back to England! We took our suitcases out of the back of the taxi and walked into the reception area of the building. There was a group of people already in the hallway with cases everywhere, and some people were greeting each other as if they had already met previously. We later learned that the building was used not only by international students, but those from all around the island too. For many students, it was a chance to move out of the family home, just like in England, and try to gain a bit of independence. So a lot of the students stayed here throughout their time at university, which is how many of the people we saw that first day already knew each other.

We were handed a huge bundle of paper, told to read it and sign the back page. Obviously the entire document was in Spanish, it was so detailed and the writing was so tiny, Cat and I just looked at each other, turned to the back page and signed. As we waited in the queue to hand it in at Reception, I flicked back through the pages. I noticed a word that looked suspiciously like the English word 'asbestos', and pointed it out to Cat. "Hmm", she said giving a nervous laugh, "interesting!" As we stood in line, we noticed a sign on the wall next to the lift had the same 'asbestos' looking word, only this time it was in red.

"It's fine", I said, "just don't touch the walls!"

What followed was to be the best year of my life. Puerto Rico is the most beautiful island; full of culture and history, with its own unique identity; it is a little taste of paradise. A paradise island with amazing beaches and plenty of rum! I had the time of my life. We were supposed to treat our time there exactly the same as if we were still studying back in England. We attended the University of Puerto Rico and I chose the Literature and History courses that looked most interesting and relevant to my American Studies course at Warwick. Although I was there to study, I was so relaxed and happy all the time, Andreas called me every other day to begin with, then after a couple of months he started to call every day. I missed him so much, but with every week that passed I knew it wouldn't be long until I saw him again. He was very supportive, and made sure I wasn't sitting pining over him, but was instead making the most of my time away. Very soon after I arrived there, he and Cat's brother Eamonn booked flights to come and see us at the end of February the following year, and I couldn't wait for him to come over and see my new home.

While I was there, I made the most amazing friends from all over the world. Studying on the beach, getting drenched in tropical rainfall then drying off in ten minutes in the sun once the rain had stopped, and then of course there was all that rum! I also really enjoyed how complicated the politics of the island were and still are, it made for a perfect topic to write my dissertation on, as the island is part of the American Commonwealth, but is not a an American State. Complications arise as the people of Puerto Rico are American citizens and hold American passports, however, not all American laws apply to the island, and on top of this, the island has many additional independent laws that are not regulated by the United States. Some people on the island are very satisfied with the status of Commonwealth, they enjoy being part of the fast American culture, as well as embracing the relaxed atmosphere and traditions of the Caribbean, but there are even more islanders who are very unhappy with it. Of these, some would prefer Puerto Rico to become America's 51st State, while others would love to see the Island completely independent from America. They consider the island to be trapped in a colonial limbo, and want to break free from the hold America has over them. This Independence movement is particularly strong amongst the students, and so I was able to do lots of research for my dissertation while I was there by participating in many discussions and demonstrations with my friends who were part of the movement. I was also able to attend debates between political party leaders, and I even managed to organise a one on one interview with a member of the Independence Party a few days before I left the island in May to return to England.

The first four months before I flew home for Christmas passed so quickly, and although I was looking forward so much to seeing my family and Andreas, I was absolutely dreading the scan that I was due to have while I was home. What if the cancer was back? I knew I wouldn't be allowed to return to Puerto Rico to finish my year, and it was times like these I grew increasingly angry with the disease, even in the sunshine with the heat beaming down on my face there was still a black cloud hanging over me. As my flight home approached, I knew that if this was the only time I would have on the island, I couldn't spoil it for myself by panicking about what waited for me back at home, so during a week's break from classes to celebrate Thanksgiving, my friends and I booked an all-inclusive week in the Dominican Republic. It cost next to nothing for Cat and I as the exchange rate was fantastic, we ate and drank and danced for the entire week, I have never felt so free, so happy. I made sure I didn't waste a second, if I was to spend another six months trapped in a hospital I wasn't going to mope around while I was here!

Once we had returned to Puerto Rico, Cat and I started to organise our flights home. It turned out to be cheaper to fly to New York and get a connecting flight on to London, rather than paying for a direct flight. "Shall we just stay in

New York for a few days, before we fly home?" Cat asked excitedly, "do a bit of Christmas shopping while we're there?"

"That's a fantastic idea!" I said. Cat and I are a terrible influence on each other, once we have an idea, no matter how expensive it may prove to be, if it involves the sun, rum, or shopping, neither of us will back down and be sensible. We'll each convince the other that it won't turn out to be as expensive as we may think, and this time we came to the conclusion that people would appreciate their Christmas presents that little bit more if they knew they came from New York! We immediately booked the flights and so straight away had to pay extra money for a little hotel to stay in for a few days only a few blocks away from Fifth Avenue. It wasn't until a few days before we were due to fly into JFK, I was packing my clothes away and realised my entire wardrobe consisted of bikinis, skirts and tiny tops—not entirely appropriate attire to be walking around New York in, in the middle of December, where it was apparently now snowing. I wondered where you would buy coats and boots from on a Caribbean island, where their winter is warmer than our summer! So Cat and I spent our last few days roaming Puerto Rico for some winter wear. Of course, the only places we could find anything to keep us warm were the big American shops—the most expensive shops! Walking around the stores, I was so excited at the thought of shopping in New York in the snow before flying home to see everyone, but once again Cat and I had succeeded in encouraging each other to spend a small fortune, this time on an entire new wardrobe each!

Leaving for the airport was quite sad, some of our friends had completed their studies in Puerto Rico and were returning to their home countries for good. Saying goodbye to some of them was heartbreaking, and they all wished me luck with my scans and the results. How funny I thought later as I sat on the plane getting ready for take off, these friends I have made from across the other side of the world, people I don't even speak the same language as have become so much closer to me, than people I grew up with. I worried I wouldn't speak to them again, that such friendships would be dispersed by distance. But I needn't have worried, with the internet and social networks, we speak so often, even now three years later, it's like we were only all together, partying and sunbathing with each other a few weeks ago.

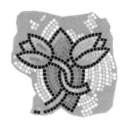

I was so happy to see Andreas again, I spent every moment I could with him, before I had to leave him again, we had a great few weeks together. But my scan results were looming, and that black cloud was threatening to rain. Again, Andreas offered to come with me to the consultation and I wanted him there with me, I wanted him to hold my hand. After being so independent and living on the other side of the world, where the people spoke a different language, it was strange to feel so vulnerable again. We traveled up to London, late of course, and in silence. He tried hard to keep my mind off the appointment, but I was terrified I wouldn't be returning to Puerto Rico the following week. We weren't waiting long for my name to be called, and I was shaking as we walked into the consultation room. Dr Whelan asked the usual questions, 'how are you?' 'Do you feel anything unusual?' Then he asked how Puerto Rico had been. I told him what a fantastic time I was having, and how I couldn't wait to go back, and he replied, "Well, the good weather obviously agrees with you, because your scans are completely clear. Go away and enjoy the rest of your time there!" I could have kissed him, the relief I felt was unimaginable, and I couldn't stop crying. Andreas gave me the biggest cuddle outside on the stairwell, I was so glad to be going back, to be able to carry on my life, to be normal!

So I went back to the Caribbean full of excitement and so relaxed. As soon as I landed and arrived back at 'Torre Del Norte', my friends who also had returned for another term of studies all asked straight away how I had got on at the hospital, their genuine delight and relief struck me when I shared my good news. I had so much to look forward to, plus Andreas and Eamonn were due to fly out and see us for just over a week at the end of February, and my mum came to visit for three weeks in April, before I returned for good in May.

I have so many fantastic memories of that year, I know I'll never have an experience like that again, and I'm so grateful it wasn't cut short by the disease. From being rescued from a broken lift by firemen to watching Ricky Martin on stage on the beach, seeing a man climb a palm tree with his hands and feet to get some coconuts to sell us, to camping on the beach to watch the most beautiful sunrise in the morning, there wasn't a single bad moment the entire time we were there. Andreas coming over with Eamonn was the icing on the cake! We were so keen to show them our new home, introduce them to our new friends and give them a little insight into our way of life, which I have to be honest mainly consisted of sunbathing and drinking the rum, but there is one night that stands out in particular . . .

We took them to a little bar at the end of our road, where the alcohol was extremely cheap. The Puerto Ricans are very generous with their measures, so we tried to warn the boys to take it slowly, but of course they didn't listen, they thought they could handle it and told us not to worry.

The following day we had arranged to take them to a tiny neighbouring island called Culebra, which is Spanish for 'snake', where one of the beaches had been voted the second most beautiful in the world. The island is absolutely breathtaking, with white sandy beaches and clear water, you can see straight down to the seabed. When you go snorkeling, even the fish are friendly as they swim around you and tickle your skin, I could have stayed there forever. We wanted them to be able to spend as much time there as possible, it was our little paradise and I wanted Andreas to share it with me. So we told the boys not to drink too much as we had an early start, and we weren't going to wait around for them while thy nursed their hangovers! When we reached the bar, we noticed they were selling a particular drink called a 'Wasikuki', and it was lethal. It contained seven different types of alcohol, but was so tooty fruity, it just tasted like a tropical fruit drink, there was no way you could detect the alcohol. "Go easy!" I warned Eamonn as I watched him knocking back his first Wasikuki of the evening.

"Leave it out! It's just like fruit juice! I'm getting another one!" He replied.

"Ok!" I said, "but we're going to Culebra in the morning, and we're flying over there in a tiny tin can plane, you really don't want to be feeling sick when that takes off!" I warned him. He just shrugged and walked away. A little later, Andreas said he was feeling tired, and wanted to get to bed so he was feeling fresh for the plane in the morning. So we went back to the hotel he and Eamonn were staying at, while Cat stayed at the bar with her brother.

"Make sure he doesn't drink too much more of that!" I said as we were leaving, "you know how it takes everyone down", I giggled as we looked over towards the bar where

Eamonn was standing, ordering yet another Wasikuki with one of our friends trying to persuade him that perhaps a rum and coke would be a better idea! Andreas and I got back to the hotel and packed our bags ready to spend a couple of days in Culebra, I couldn't wait to get there, I knew he would love it just as much as I did. We snuggled up in front of the TV as I described how beautiful it was over there, and we drifted off to sleep.

I woke in the middle of the night to use the loo, and as I walked over to the bathroom, I looked over at Eamonn's bed noticing that it was still empty. Hmm, I thought as I closed the bathroom door, we have to be up in three hours and he still isn't home, I hope he's with Cat getting some sleep! As I turned the light out in the bathroom, I sleepily shuffled back to bed, and pulled the covers over my head. I was just drifting back off to sleep when the front door to the room flung open. It was Eamonn, absolutely smashed. He stood in the doorway with his hands raised to the sky, seemingly triumphant that he had found his way home, "You alright mate?" Andreas asked blinking from the light coming in through the doorway.

"I AM . . . THE WASIKUKI KING!" Eamonn proclaimed at the top of his voice for all of Puerto Rico to hear. With that he launched himself into the air and flew across the room towards his bed, which was beside the wall on the opposite side of the room to Andreas and I. Unfortunately, in his jubilation at being the 'Wasikuki King' he overestimated the distance between himself and his bed and crashed head first into the wall, then slid down towards the floor and was jammed in between the bed and the wall with his legs protruding up towards the ceiling. Andreas and I sat up in bed staring in astonishment over at the two legs sticking out from behind the covers, not really knowing what to say. And that's where Eamonn stayed, for the rest of the night. Needless to say, the 'Wasikuki King' wasn't too happy being woken up three hours later and being told to pack quickly as we were heading for the airport, but I had warned him!

We had a fantastic time in Culebra and the rest of the week flew by, soon it was time for the boys to leave. I was sad to wave Andreas off at the airport, but I only had a couple of months left in the sun, so tried hard not to feel too down and looked forward to mum coming over a few weeks later.

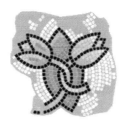

If it hadn't been for Andreas, I'm not sure I would have come home from Puerto Rico. It was absolutely gorgeous, and the people were so lovely. The culture and politics are so complicated, intricate and unique that despite it being, at face value, just a tiny island off the coast of Florida, it truly has it's own identity and a huge personality! I was so upset when I left, and absolutely devastated to be saying goodbye to some people, but I should have known that true friends really do stick around forever. In fact, I have since popped over to Milan to see one friend who was from Italy, and am really looking forward to flying out to Indiana in the States next year to attend another friend's wedding, and most of the girls I met over there have been to stay in London with Cat and I since. If only I had known that all this was to come when I was fretting over losing my friends all those years ago. How funny that they all literally live down the road from me, and yet I see people living on the other side of the world more often, I guess true friendship doesn't see colour, race or differences in culture and language. I'm going back to Puerto Rico next year with Andreas for a little holiday, and I can't wait; I can't wait to feel the sun on my face, to dance on the beach, and be with all my lovely friends again, it really is a little taste of paradise.

As soon as I touched down in London, reality hit. I got home, excited to see everyone; waiting for me was a pile of letters and appointments from hospital, all lined up for the following month. Urghh, I thought, I want to run back to Puerto Rico! But I had no time to feel sorry for myself, my friends Katharine, Becky, Louise and Justine wanted to meet up for a drink, and to hear all about my Caribbean adventures. I had a shock walking into the pub and being charged three times the amount for half the alcohol that I was used to in Puerto Rico, but as much as I missed the island, I was so happy to be surrounded by my lovely girlfriends!

A month later it was time to pick up my results. This time I was really confident. I felt really good, after the year away I was the fittest and healthiest I had ever been, and I felt really relaxed. It was the one and only time I had ever been, not only on time, but actually early for a consultation, and I sat in the waiting room with Andreas flicking through a magazine, "You ok honey?" he asked, rubbing my back.

"Yeah, I'm fine actually," surprised at my own reply, "I'm going to be fine!" We sat in the waiting room until it was time to hear my results. I breezed into the consultation room, and smiled at Dr Whelan "Wow!" he said, "you're tanned! You look really good!"

"I feel good", I replied, as I sat down in front of him. He didn't waste anytime giving me the results, and I smiled at him expecting him to tell me to go away and come back in six months.

"It's come back Natasha", he said. I couldn't believe what I was hearing,

"But I feel so well", desperate for him to realise he had made a mistake.

"It's in your liver again, but the tumours are in a slightly different place. I think we should try the Radio Frequency Ablation therapy again, the same treatment we gave you on your liver a couple of years ago".

"But it hasn't worked, has it?" Andreas asked, "why has it come back?"

"The treatment did work", Dr Whelan explained, "these tumours are not in the same site as the previous ones, and the rest of your scans are clear, so I don't think it warrants another dose of chemotherapy, unless you want chemo, just to be safe?"

"Er no!" I answered, "let's try the RFA treatment again. I guess it's promising if the tumours are in a different place now. Christ! I just need a complete body transplant, don't I?" I tried to joke. My consultant laughed as he gathered some paperwork together and prepared to get this next set of treatment in motion.

So I had more RFA treatment. I worried again about my studies, but at least this time I was in the middle of a summer break, I could have the treatment and recover before it was time to start my final year at Warwick. Despite this new thorn on my rose, I tried hard to stop my bud from withering under the unrelenting pressure of this disease. The treatment went well, and this time I knew what to expect and knew how long I would be in pain for afterwards. I was keen to get it over and done with as soon as possible, as I was approaching the final and most important year of my degree, I couldn't let anything get in the way, I had worked too hard to throw it all away now! Once again, I picked myself up, dusted myself off and got on with life. I carried on with university, and travelled home each weekend as I had a little

Saturday job in a restaurant in London, and it also gave me a chance to see Andreas regularly after having been away from him for so long! After the summer, I completed my dissertation on the political situation in Puerto Rico, which brought back so many beautiful memories, and so now I had the chance to focus completely on my final exams. I was excited to be coming to the end of my studies, but quite nervous as the grown-up world of work loomed, I wanted to do as well as possible, to give myself the best possible chance of getting a good job, and enjoy a comfortable life. But I had one more scan between now and those exams, I couldn't fall at the last hurdle, and I knew that if I needed any more chemo I wouldn't be able to finish my degree, well, not that year anyway. So I was terrified walking into the consultation room six months later the day my next set of results were due. I had felt so well last time and it had been bad news, so despite feeling great and positive again, I knew that I couldn't assume what these results would say.

It was bad news again, it had returned in my liver yet again, this was the third time it had been diagnosed in my liver, the fifth time in all and so Dr Whelan suggested chemotherapy. Although the tiny tumours, again, were in a slightly different place than before, Dr Whelan pointed out that more and more tumours were appearing at quite a regular rate now, so there was a huge chance that if I had RFA therapy again, in six months time when I was back for my next set of scans, I would be in exactly the same situation again. But I couldn't do it, I only had three months left at university.

"Let me have RFA therapy just one more time, let me finish my studies and if it's back again in six months, I'll come back for chemo, at least by then I'll hopefully have my degree". My consultant knew how hard I had battled for my education since this whole nightmare began, It was the only thing really that kept me going, it gave me a focus, a goal to reach, and stopped me from giving up and giving in to this poison. So he agreed.

Again, my professors at Warwick were so understanding, and compassionate. They wanted me to do well too, so were very patient with me handing in my final assessed pieces of work for the year, and any practise exam papers we were set. I had a lovely Spanish teacher that year, her name was Consuelo, she was so kind and encouraging, and as my treatment got underway she was just happy to see me in her class with or without any assessed work I was meant to have completed! It took a lot of pressure off me, and allowed me to concentrate on getting better first, then I could focus on my work, and finally get that degree! "I knew I should have stayed in Puerto Rico!" I said to mum before I went in for the RFA operation, "I was completely clear the entire time I was there, but I've been diagnosed twice in 12 months now I'm home!" She kissed me on the forehead as I was wheeled in for my anaesthetic with Andreas by my side. As I felt the familiar feeling of the anaesthetic being fed through the vein in my arm and a wave of drowsiness consumed me, I struggled to pull myself up in the bed and called to Andreas for a kiss, but it was too late. I was asleep.

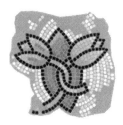

That was two years ago now, I have been completely clear since, and haven't taken a single second for granted. I graduated from Warwick with a 2.1 in Comparative American Studies, and have been working hard ever since. I know it will come back eventually but I can't let it get me down. This isn't a death sentence for me, and although it may be what causes my rose to whither in the end, it certainly hasn't stopped the bud from blossoming! It is so important to grab life by the balls. Even if cancer or disease has never been a thorn on your rose, something you have never even thought about, you must still live every second as if it's your last. We all go through tough times, we all struggle, we all draw the short straw at some point whether it's in heath, wealth, love or work. But you mustn't despair if your rose seems to be wilting, it may just need a little sunlight. My sunlight is my friends Katharine, Rebecca, Louise, Justine and Cat, and all the amazing people I have met on my travels along the way. My sunlight is my family, my incredible mum, my brother and my nan,—and grandad, who smiles down on us everyday. My sunlight is Andreas.

So Shall It Be In The End

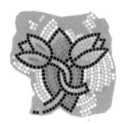

I have so many dreams; so many plans for how I want my life to work out. Sometimes I get frustrated that things aren't happening fast enough, while other times I worry that I'm going to run out of time. I wonder if the disease will get me before I achieve all the things I want to.

I know that my experiences and challenges over the last ten years have made me stronger, more confident, independent and focused. But I also know that I wouldn't be who I am today without my family. Whenever I feel low, worried or I'm just feeling sorry for myself, they're always around to pick me up.

I know that this will never go away. It will always be hanging over my shoulder, and sometimes just this thought alone gets me down. Most days though, it actually gives me the drive I need to chase my dreams, to succeed, to push for things I otherwise might have been too scared to reach for. As I sit here waiting for my consultant's call with my latest scan results, I smile at all the aspirations I have and the possibilities that lie ahead of me. The last 25 years have certainly been a bumpy ride, the thorns on my rose have caused, often, unbearable pain. But the bud is blooming, and as life passes, the flower looks more and more beautiful everyday.

I have to go now, the phone's ringing . . .

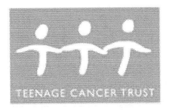

Teenage Cancer Trust understands what teenagers need to fight cancer.

At a time when your body is changing, your social life is everything and you're still trying to figure out who you are, getting cancer can seem like an impossible blow to take. But thanks to Teenage Cancer Trust, thousands of teenagers are taking it, and coming out fighting.

Teenage Cancer Trust doesn't believe teenagers should have to stop being teenagers, just because they have cancer. So they fund and build specialist units for young people in NHS hospitals. These units bring teenagers with cancer together so they can be treated alongside each other, by cancer experts, in an environment that's tailored to meet their needs.

Teenage Cancer Trust units aren't like ordinary cancer wards. Everything about them has been designed to give teenagers the best possible quality of life and chances of survival.

To find out more visit **teenagecancertrust.org** email tct@teenagecancertrust.org or call 020 7612 0370

Teenage Cancer Trust is a registered charity in England & Wales (1062559); Scotland (SCO39757)

Printed in Great Britain
by Amazon.co.uk, Ltd.,
Marston Gate.